T0226965

Extracorporeal Membrane Oxygenation

Editors

NITIN PURI
MICHAEL BARAM
NICHOLAS C. CAVAROCCHI

CRITICAL CARE CLINICS

www.criticalcare.theclinics.com

Consulting Editor
JOHN A. KELLUM

October 2017 • Volume 33 • Number 4

ELSEVIER

1600 John F. Kennedy Boulevard • Suite 1800 • Philadelphia, Pennsylvania, 19103-2899

http://www.theclinics.com

CRITICAL CARE CLINICS Volume 33, Number 4
October 2017 ISSN 0749-0704, ISBN-13: 978-0-323-54658-4

Editor: Katie Pfaff
Developmental Editor: Casey Potter

Critical Care Clinics (ISSN: 0749-0704) is published quarterly by Elsevier Inc., 360 Park Avenue South, New York, NY 10010-1710. Months of issue are January, April, July, and October. Business and Editorial Offices: 1600 John F. Kennedy Blvd., Suite 1800, Philadelphia, PA 19103-2899. Customer Service Office: 6277 Sea Harbor Drive, Orlando, FL 32887-4800. Periodicals postage paid at New York, NY and additional mailing offices. Subscription prices are $221.00 per year for US individuals, $584.00 per year for US institution, $100.00 per year for US students and residents, $263.00 per year for Canadian individuals, $732.00 per year for Canadian institutions, $309.00 per year for international individuals, $732.00 per year for international institutions and $150.00 per year for Canadian and foreign students/ residents. To receive student/resident rate, orders must be accompanied by name of affiliated institution, date of term, and the signature of program/residency coordinator on institution letterhead. Orders will be billed at individual rate until proof of status is received. Foreign air speed delivery is included in all *Clinics* subscription prices. All prices are subject to change without notice. POSTMASTER: Send address changes to *Critical Care Clinics*, Elsevier Periodicals Customer Service, 11830 Westline Industrial Drive, St. Louis, MO 63146. **Customer Service: 1-800-654-2452 (US). From outside of the US, call 1-314-447-8871. Fax: 1-314-447-8029. E-mail: journalscustomerservice-usa@ elsevier.com (for print support) or journalsonlinesupport-usa@elsevier.com (for online support).**

Reprints. For copies of 100 or more of articles in this publication, please contact the Commercial Reprints Department, Elsevier Inc., 360 Park Avenue South, New York, NY 10010-1710. Tel.: 212-633-3874; Fax: 212-633-3820; E-mail: reprints@elsevier.com.

Critical Care Clinics is also published in Spanish by Editorial Inter-Medica, Junin 917, 1er A, 1113, Buenos Aires, Argentina.

Critical Care Clinics is covered in *MEDLINE/PubMed (Index Medicus), EMBASE/Excerpta Medica, Current Concepts/ Clinical Medicine, ISI/BIOMED, and Chemical Abstracts.*

Contributors

CONSULTING EDITOR

JOHN A. KELLUM, MD, MCCM
Professor of Critical Care Medicine, Medicine, Bioengineering and Clinical & Translational Science, Director, Center for Critical Care Nephrology, Vice Chair for Research, Department of Critical Care Medicine, University of Pittsburgh School of Medicine, Pittsburgh, Pennsylvania

EDITORS

NITIN PURI, MD
Program Director, Division of Critical Care Medicine, Associate Professor, Department of Medicine, Cooper University Hospital, Camden, New Jersey

MICHAEL BARAM, MD
Fellowship Program Director for Pulmonary and Critical Care, Korman Lung Center, Associate Professor, Division of Pulmonary and Critical Care Medicine, Department of Medicine, Thomas Jefferson University, Philadelphia, Pennsylvania

NICHOLAS C. CAVAROCCHI, MD
Director, Cardiac Critical Care, Professor, Division of Cardiothoracic Surgery, Department of Surgery, Thomas Jefferson University, Philadelphia, Pennsylvania

AUTHORS

BHARAT AWSARE, MD, FCCP
Division of Pulmonary and Critical Care Medicine, Department of Medicine, Thomas Jefferson University, Philadelphia, Pennsylvania

MICHAEL BARAM, MD
Fellowship Program Director for Pulmonary and Critical Care, Korman Lung Center, Associate Professor, Division of Pulmonary and Critical Care Medicine, Department of Medicine, Thomas Jefferson University, Philadelphia, Pennsylvania

MONIKA F. CARDONA, BSN, RN
ECMO and CRRT Nurse Manager, Medical University of South Carolina, Charleston, South Carolina

NICHOLAS C. CAVAROCCHI, MD
Director, Cardiac Critical Care, Professor, Division of Cardiothoracic Surgery, Department of Surgery, Thomas Jefferson University, Philadelphia, Pennsylvania

HEIDI J. DALTON, MD
Director, Department of Pediatrics, Adult and Pediatric ECMO, INOVA Fairfax Medical Campus, Inova Fairfax Hospital, Falls Church, Virginia; Professor, Department of Clinical Surgery, The George Washington University, Washington, DC

EDWARD M. DARLING, MS, CCP
Associate Professor, Department of Cardiovascular Perfusion, SUNY Upstate Medical University, Syracuse, New York

DAVID C. FITZGERALD, MPH, CCP
Clinical Coordinator, Division of Cardiovascular Perfusion, MUSC College of Health Professions, Medical University of South Carolina, Charleston, South Carolina

JUSTIN HERMAN, MD
Division of Pulmonary and Critical Care Medicine, Department of Medicine, Thomas Jefferson University, Philadelphia, Pennsylvania

HITOSHI HIROSE, MD, PhD
Professor of Surgery, Department of Cardiothoracic Surgery, Thomas Jefferson University, Philadelphia, Pennsylvania

CHRISTOPHER LOREN JENKS, MD
Clinical Instructor, Department of Pediatrics, Section of Critical Care Medicine, Cardiac Intensive Care Unit, Baylor College of Medicine, Texas Children's Hospital, Houston, Texas

JULIA JONES-AKHTAREKHAVARI, BSN, RN, CCRN
Mechanical Circulatory Support Manager, Department of Mechanical Circulatory Support, Gill Heart & Vascular Institute, UK HealthCare, Lexington, Kentucky

CHRISTOPHER S. KING, MD, FACP, FCCP
Medical Director, Advanced Lung Disease and Lung Transplantation Critical Care, Department of Medicine, Inova Fairfax Hospital, Falls Church, Virginia

WALTER K. KRAFT, MD
Associate Professor, Director, Clinical Research Unit and Division of Clinical Pharmacology, Department of Pharmacology and Experimental Therapeutics, Thomas Jefferson University, Philadelphia, Pennsylvania

KATHLEEN M. LAMB, MD
Division of Vascular Surgery and Endovascular Therapy, Hospital of the University of Pennsylvania, Philadelphia, Pennsylvania

KYLE C. NIZIOLEK, MD, EMT-P
Critical Care Medicine Fellow, Critical Care Medicine, Cooper University Health Care, Camden, New Jersey

ERIK C. OSBORN, MD
Colonel, United States Army, Medical Corps, Pulmonary Critical Care Sleep Medicine, Fort Belvoir Community Hospital, Fort Belvoir, Virginia; Assistant Professor, Uniformed Services University of the Health Sciences, Bethesda, Maryland

MICHELLE PEAHOTA, PharmD
Advanced Practice Clinical Pharmacist, Department of Pharmacy, Thomas Jefferson University, Philadelphia, Pennsylvania

HARRISON T. PITCHER, MD
Associate Professor of Surgery, Department of Cardiothoracic Surgery, Thomas Jefferson University, Philadelphia, Pennsylvania

THOMAS J. PRESTON, BS, CCP, FPP
Co-Owner, Innovative ECMO Concepts, Inc, Arcadia, Oklahoma

LAKSHMI RAMAN, MD
Assistant Professor, Department of Pediatrics, Section Critical Care Medicine, The University of Texas Southwestern Medical Center, Children's Medical Center at Dallas, Dallas, Texas

AVIRAL ROY, MBBS
Critical Care Fellow, Critical Care Medicine, Cooper University Health Care, Camden, New Jersey

LIAM RYAN, MD
Department of Cardiothoracic Surgery, Inova Fairfax Hospital, Falls Church, Virginia

AMI G. SHAH, PharmD
Department of Pharmacy, Thomas Jefferson University, Philadelphia, Pennsylvania

RAMESH SINGH, MD
Department of Cardiothoracic Surgery, Inova Fairfax Hospital, Falls Church, Virginia

BRANDI N. THOMA, PharmD
Advanced Practice Clinical Pharmacist, Department of Pharmacy, Thomas Jefferson University, Philadelphia, Pennsylvania

THOMAS A. TRIBBLE, AA
Mechanical Circulatory Support Specialist, Department of Mechanical Circulatory Support, Gill Heart & Vascular Institute, UK HealthCare, University of Kentucky, Lexington, Kentucky

JOSEPH B. ZWISCHENBERGER, MD, FACS, FCCP
Johnston-Wright Professor, Chairman, Department of Surgery, University of Kentucky College of Medicine, Lexington, Kentucky

Contents

(ARDS). Part of the current critical care knowledge base must include an understanding of how extracorporeal membrane oxygenation fits into the paradigm of ARDS management without using it as a "salvage therapy." This article provides a basic understanding of the evolution of ARDS to multiple organ dysfunction syndrome, recognizing benefits and limits of rescue therapies, indications and contraindications of extracorporeal membrane oxygenation, and coordination of care for severe respiratory failure.

Venoarterial extracorporeal membrane oxygenation is a rescue therapy in patients with severe cardiopulmonary failure. Often, cannulation is done emergently and the femoral vessels are most readily accessible for venous and arterial access. Unfortunately, complications with arterial femoral access can lead to devastating complications, primarily related to limb ischemia. A coordinated protocol of diligent limb examination by trained intensive care unit staff, near infrared spectroscopy monitoring of limbs, and placement of a distal perfusion catheter at the time of femoral cannulation or when signs of ischemia develop, can lead to successful limb salvage.

Extracorporeal life support is a modified form of cardiopulmonary bypass. Experience in extracorporeal membrane oxygenation (ECMO) has come largely from the neonatal population. Most centers have transitioned the ECMO pumps from roller pumps to centrifugal technology. Modes of support include venovenous for respiratory support and venoarterial for cardiac support. "Awake" ECMO is the trend, with extubation and tracheostomy on the rise. Fluid overload is common and managed with diuretics or hemofiltration. Nutrition is important and provided enterally or via total parenteral nutrition. Overall survival for pediatric cardiac and respiratory ECMO has remained at approximately 50% to 60%.

Extracorporeal membrane oxygenation (ECMO) is a life-saving technique when patients require pulmonary and/or cardiac support for days to weeks for recovery, bridge to decision, or transplantation. Due to complications associated with ECMO, it is best to stay on ECMO as little time as necessary. Foremost is weaning from ECMO, but the post-ECMO period recapitulates the entire field of critical care. Identified issues include (1) potential for systemic inflammatory response syndrome after decannulation; (2) post-ECMO complications, such as deep vein thrombosis, wounds, renal failure, and stroke; (3) delirium; (4) posttraumatic stress disorder; (5) rehabilitation; and (6) end of life.

x

Extracorporeal Membrane Oxygenation
CRITICAL CARE CLINICS

THE CLINICS ARE AVAILABLE ONLINE!
Access your subscription at:
www.theclinics.com

Preface

Extracorporeal Membrane Oxygenation

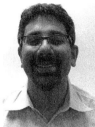 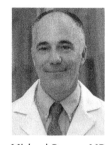 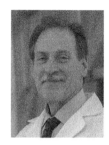

Nitin Puri, MD   Michael Baram, MD   Nicholas C. Cavarocchi, MD

Editors

Over the years, there have been many innovations that have come and gone. It is not often that a single idea dramatically changes how critical care is delivered. Since the era of the Vietnam War, Intensivists have been dealing with acute respiratory distress syndrome (formally known as Da Nang lung, adult respiratory distress, and others) and cardiogenic shock, but with recent developments in extracorporeal membrane oxygenation (ECMO), ECMO is able to sustain life to give these critically ill patients an opportunity to heal. Just as importantly, systems had to evolve to facilitate transfer of critically ill patients, equipment had to be developed to fly heart-lung equipment between facilities, protocols for transport had to be created, and (gasp) pulmonologists had to cooperate with cardiothoracic surgeons. ECMO support has required hospitals to either commit tremendous resources to establish ECMO programs or align with ECMO centers to refer these patients to hospitals that do have ECMO support. Over the past decade, ECMO programs grew at different rates, with different components, and with different styles. This issue of *Critical Care Clinics* had contributors from multiple ECMO sites to help share ideas that have proven successful. The editors would like to thank all the contributors for their time to compose this issue and for their dedication to ECMO services.

Nitin Puri, MD
Division of Critical Care Medicine
Department of Medicine
Cooper University Hospital
One Cooper Plaza
Camden, NJ 08103, USA

Crit Care Clin 33 (2017) xi–xii
http://dx.doi.org/10.1016/j.ccc.2017.07.002
0749-0704/17/© 2017 Published by Elsevier Inc.

criticalcare.theclinics.com

Michael Baram, MD
Korman Lung Center
Thomas Jefferson University
834 Walnut Street, Suite 650
Philadelphia, PA 19107, USA

Nicholas C. Cavarocchi, MD
Thomas Jefferson University
1025 Walnut Street, Suite 605
Philadelphia, PA 19073, USA

E-mail addresses:
purimon@gmail.com (N. Puri)
michael.baram@jefferson.edu (M. Baram)
Nicholas.cavarocchi@jefferson.edu (N.C. Cavarocchi)

Introduction to Extracorporeal Membrane Oxygenation

 CrossMark

Nicholas C. Cavarocchi, MD

KEYWORDS

• ECMO • Multidisciplinary • Team building

KEY POINTS

• Extracorporeal membrane oxygenation (ECMO) has a long history of providing lifesaving support to patients.
• ECMO has evolved in application over time.
• Utility of ECMO requires a full team of trained professionals.
• Initiation of ECMO requires an organized, preplanned, coordinated effort.

INTRODUCTION

Suddenly there was a cardiac arrest on the hospital lobby floor and I recognized it was the hospital painter, a familiar face. The resuscitation process had begun. An unfamiliar voice from behind hollered out, "Secure the airway, lines in, and begin effective chest compressions! … the team will setup the heart-lung machine for extracorporeal membrane oxygenation" (ECMO). As a surgical intern, I blindly followed the orders, not having any idea about what we were planning to do next. Somehow over the next minutes I began my surgical career, cutting down on the groin and performing cannulation of the femoral vessels for cardiopulmonary bypass. I was overwhelmed at my success but not willing to ask the most important question: What is next? The chief calmly spoke out: "Now we have time to think." What a novel idea in the middle of the lobby on the floor with blood everywhere. I listened how he rationalized that the diagnosis was a pulmonary embolus. We proceeded to the operating room and performed the embolectomy. The diagnosis was correct; the procedure went well; our patient survived intact. It worked. I learned that day that ECMO provided respiratory and cardiac support but did not treat the underlying pathologic condition. It allowed us time to think.

It was 1979 and I was hooked on extracorporeal life support (ECLS).

The author does not have any commercial or financial conflicts of interest or funding sources related to this article.
Division of Cardiothoracic Surgery, Department of Surgery, Thomas Jefferson University, 1025 Walnut Street, Suite 605, Philadelphia, PA 19073, USA
E-mail address: Nicholas.Cavarocchi@jefferson.edu

HISTORY

The question remains: Does ECMO really work? In 1979, the first randomized controlled data trial was published by Zapol and colleagues[1] in *The Journal of the American Medical Association* and concluded that there was no survival benefit to ECMO, with a high complication rate. From this article, ECMO sustained a significant setback but the enthusiasm continued through observational reports. In 1994 Morris and colleagues[2] published the second randomized trial, comparing pressure control inverse ratio ventilation versus extracorporeal carbon dioxide removal in adult respiratory distress syndrome (ARDS) and demonstrated survival of less than 10% with no significance differences. ECLS had suffered another major setback. These randomized trials are now recognized to have archaic ECMO technology, nonvetted treatment protocols, poor ventilator management, and high complication rates for infections and severe bleeding complications. Both the Zapol[1] and the Morris[2] trials have little relevance to current ECMO regimens.

Through the 1990s, there was particular interest by select groups in the United States and the United Kingdom in treating ARDS, pneumonias, and congenital disorders. The new era of the ECMO paradigm shift began at the turn of the millennia with the Conventional Ventilatory Support versus Extracorporeal Membrane Oxygenation for Severe Adult Respiratory Failure (CESAR) trial, the H1N1 influenza epidemic, new technology, and management protocols.[3,4] The CESAR trial was designed as an intent-to-treat trial comparing conventional ventilation with ECMO for severe ARDS at a referral center in the United Kigdom.[3] The primary outcome measures demonstrated a reduction in death or severe disability in the ECMO group (37% vs 53%); the secondary outcomes showed decreased ventilator time, length of intensive care unit (ICU) stay, blood usage, and cost of health care. The findings supported that lung rest via ECMO was feasible and that ARDS should be managed at tertiary care centers. The H1N1 epidemic, which began in Australia, showed the world that ECMO could be used by tertiary centers during high-volume crises. The Australian lead set the framework for the H1N1 epidemic as it spread across the hemispheres. They demonstrated a 71% survival in patients who failed conventional medical treatment of ARDS secondary to H1N1.[4] This sentinel article demonstrated advances in technology of blood oxygenators, circulatory pumps, and intravascular cannula design. This new ECMO technology allowed for longer circuit runs with fewer complications. Traditionally, prolonged ECMO runs were limited by hemolysis, bleeding, and infections. The advantages of centrifugal pumps were less hemolysis, heparin, and transfusions requirements resulting in fewer circuit-related complications. The advantages of new membrane oxygenators included increased longevity, less blood trauma, and improved gas exchange. It was too late for randomization; the door was open, and the interest was ongoing.

Management protocols and algorithms were nonexistence in 2005. The Extracorporeal Life Support Organization (ELSO) created guidelines for training, staffing, and equipment. Attempts were made to control costs and reduce labor requirements.[5] There was a practical recognition that bedside circuitry needed to be affordable, reliable, simple, and transportable. Monitoring patients on ECLS in the ICU required extension to a team approach not just trained surgical specialists. This requirement is especially true with multiple patients on prolonged support. The published 2005 ELSO data showed that historically, ECMO was primarily used for congenital and pediatric diseases.[5]

PROGRAM EVOLUTION

A decade later, there has been an increase in the number of adult ECMO cases due to the improvement in equipment, renewed interest, and growth of ECMO teams.[6] The past history of ECMO has revolved around respiratory failure in neonates with sporadic adults cases; as salvage or delay to death strategy with open cutdowns or chest incisions. This resulted in being both labor and resource intensive and a complicated system. There have been decades worth of multiple techniques, technology, and management strategies that have failed along the course of time. This expansion in use has required a development of standardized approaches in critically ill ECMO patients.

The questions that developed in the ICU included the following: Was multi-organ failure reversible[7]? Could we monitor for cerebral and limb neurologic complications[8]? How do we wean patients from ECMO? Can we predict the respiratory indicators for initiation and liberation from ECMO? Over time the indications, absolute or relative contraindications, and outcome data have continued to evolve with multiple centers.

Modern-day support for respiratory and cardiac failure should provide time for treatment and recovery, a quick and easy system that is portable and easy to transfer. Programs should revolve around effective use of hospital resources, cost-effectiveness, and few complications and offer advanced ventricular and respiratory therapies, such as ventricular assist devices, total artificial heart, and thoracic organ transplantation.

Program development centers on 5 principles: education, standardized care, interdisciplinary team, database and modernized equipment, and monitoring devices. The educational process begins with the ICU team of perfusionists, respiratory therapist, and the nursing staff. Standardize care revolves around policies, algorithms, and order sets. The interdisciplinary team revolves around leadership, administration, nursing staff, perfusion, ICU team, respiratory therapy, surgeons, cardiologists, and pulmonologists. Modernized equipment revolves around state-of-the-art pumps and oxygenators, heparinized cannulas and tubing, and point-of-care devices, such as oximetry. It is important to realize that program development is labor and equipment intensive; it is cost prohibitive for long-term care; it must meet continuing medical education guidelines for minimum number of cases for payments while returning patients to the community.

Building a network allows easy access for other hospitals and patients to centers of excellence, with prompt feedback and eventual return of patients to their community. Planning allows for one phone call access to centers of excellence, with transportation by trained personnel either by air or ground. Patients can develop intermediate term issues revolving around sedation, sepsis, tracheotomy care, deep vein thrombosis, and neuropathies of critical illnesses. Follow-up of pulmonary functions, chest examinations, and physical and mental quality of life needs to be studied and treated by experts.

ISSUE STRUCTURE

ECMO has evolved from case reports to case series and now with randomized trials to support the benefits of ECMO.[3] Despite all the advances, there is still variation in how ECMO is used and implemented. Throughout this issue dedicated to ECMO, there are varying opinions and thoughts. These varying viewpoints were not oversights or mis-edits. Instead the editors sought input from authors across the country to be sure that this issue represents many thought leaders and not just the author's institution's bias.

The overarching goal of this issue was to educate ECMO providers of all the intraces that may not be part of their routine practice. For example, the article on vascular issues will not teach a surgeon the details of how to operate on large blood vessels, instead it attempts to explain to internists why operative closure of these sites is important. The same holds true for ventilator management; books could be written on the physiology of heart-lung-vent-ECMO interactions. Instead this issue focuses on why it is important to for ECMO patients to have intensivists manage the ventilator. As a whole, this issue highlights the complexity of ECMO patients and supports the growth of interdisciplinary teams and administrative support.

SUMMARY

The time is on us to call on personnel in the field to come up with consistent indications, contraindications, techniques, technology, and outcome in this modern era. This issue is a collection of visions of what it takes to build a program, how to maintain it, and the most current ideas and data in the field.

REFERENCES

1. Zapol WM, Snider MT, Hill JD, et al. Extracorporeal membrane oxygenation in severe acute respiratory failure: a randomized prospective study. JAMA 1979; 242(20):2193–6.
2. Morris AH, Wallace CJ, Menlove RL, et al. Randomized clinical trial of pressure-controlled inverse ratio ventilation and extracorporeal CO2 removal for adult respiratory distress syndrome. Am J Respir Crit Care Med 1994;149(2):295–305.
3. Conventional Ventilation or ECMO for Severe Adult Respiratory Failure Trial Investigators. CESAR trial: ISRCTN47279827. Available at: http://www.cesar-trial.org/. Accessed May 27, 2008.
4. The Australia and New Zealand Extracorporeal Membrane Oxygenation (ANZ ECMO) Influenza Investigators, Davies A, Jones D, Bailey M, et al. Extracorporeal membrane oxygenation for 2009 influenza A(H1N1) acute respiratory distress syndrome. JAMA 2009;302(17):1888–95.
5. ELSO guidelines for ECMO centers. Extracorporeal Life Support Organization Web site. Available at: http://www.elsonet.org/. Accessed January 1, 2016.
6. Thiagarajan RR, Barbaro RP, Rycus PT, et al. Extracorporeal Life Support Organization registry international report 2016. ASAIO J 2017;63(1):60–7.
7. Wong JK, Siow VS, Hirose H, et al. End organ recovery and survival with the QuadroxD oxygenator in adults on extracorporeal membrane oxygenation. Word J Cardiovasc Surg 2012;2:73–80.
8. Wong JK, Smith TN, Pitcher HT, et al. Cerebral and lower limb near-infrared spectroscopy in adults on extracorporeal membrane oxygenation. Artif Organs 2012; 36:659–67.

Developing an Extracorporeal Membrane Oxygenation Program

Julia Jones-Akhtarekhavari, BSN, RN, CCRN[a], Thomas A. Tribble, AA[b],
Joseph B. Zwischenberger, MD[c],*

KEYWORDS

- Patient management • Implementation • Outcomes • Multidisciplinary approach

KEY POINTS

- The Extracorporeal Life Support Organization (ELSO) has developed guidelines that outline the ideal institutional requirements for the development of an extracorporeal membrane oxygenation (ECMO) program.
- The development of an ECMO program requires institutional commitment, advanced technology and equipment, and the multidisciplinary cooperation of trained specialty personnel.
- The ELSO provides an international registry that voluntarily collects centers' individual reported data and offers clinical research support, quality assessment, and regulatory updates related to ECMO therapy.

INTRODUCTION

Extracorporeal membrane oxygenation (ECMO) is a rapidly evolving field that was developed more than 40 years ago for critically ill patients with respiratory failure. Despite other terms used, such as extracorporeal life support (ECLS), ECMO is most often used to refer to all forms of extracorporeal support if gas exchange is involved and is a form of life support for critically ill patients when traditional supportive care is no longer effective. (In this article, which refers directly to source material, the terms

Disclosure Statement: J. Jones-Akhtarekhavari and T.A. Tribble have nothing to disclose. J.B. Zwischenberger is the coinventor of a US patented double lumen catheter, often used with extracorporeal membrane oxygenation; he receives royalties from Avalon-Maquet, to which the patent is licensed.
^a Department of Mechanical Circulatory Support, Gill Heart & Vascular Institute, UK HealthCare, Pavilion A 08.261, 1000 South Limestone, Lexington, KY 40536, USA; ^b Department of Mechanical Circulatory Support, Gill Heart & Vascular Institute, UK HealthCare, University of Kentucky, 800 Rose Street, Lexington, KY 40536, USA; ^c Department of Surgery, University of Kentucky, 800 Rose Street, MN-264, Lexington, KY 40536, USA
* Corresponding author.
E-mail address: jzwis2@uky.edu

ECMO and ECLS are used interchangeably.) ECMO has also become a bridge to transplantation and a way to manage acute shock. Over the past 15 years, with the further advancement of ECMO technologies, both the need and demand for ECMO have grown, requiring the development of more ECMO centers.[1] The development of an ECMO program, however, requires institutional commitment, advanced technology and equipment, and the multidisciplinary cooperation of trained specialty personnel.

INSTITUTIONAL COMMITMENT

The Extracorporeal Life Support Organization (ELSO) has developed guidelines that outline the ideal institutional requirements for the development of an ECMO program.[2] These guidelines suggest an ECMO program is best suited to a tertiary medical center that is centrally/regionally located with a tertiary-level neonatal ICU, pediatric ICU, and/or adult ICU. The institution should also be capable of financially supporting the level of expertise required as well as managing the program's overall cost effectiveness.

Market Analysis

Before planning for the execution and implementation of an ECMO program, an institution must evaluate the regional market. It is crucial to understand the market, regional competitors, and the patient population to predict potential patient volumes and the potential for long-term sustainability.

Needs Assessment

Establishing and maintaining an ECMO program is resource intensive. Prior to initiating a program, a needs assessment is necessary to identify a facility's capability to support a program. Careful consideration must be applied to financial impact, access, and occupancy because the initiation of a program will have an impact on existing critical care services.

Primarily, the center must confirm occupancy of critical care areas allows for the addition of an ECMO program. Total length of stay and ICU length of stay for an ECLS patient are typically much longer than for patients in other specialty areas. Depending on the location of ECLS patient cohort, the addition of ECLS patients could have a negative impact on operating room (OR) throughput and access to ICU beds for non-ECLS referrals.

Self-limiting factors
1. Bed occupancy rate
2. Physician/clinical staff
3. Nursing staff

Knowledge of ECMO as a bridge therapy should be used when designing a program. Although many patients do recover, a small number may require more advanced or durable solutions. The program must be designed with an understanding of the potential for patients to bridge to additional advanced therapies, such as transplantation and ventricular assist devices. ECMO programs without these services should coordinate with centers for the transfer of these patients for consideration of ventricular assist device or transplantation candidacy.

Program Vision

Once the needs assessment and financial modeling are complete, planning for the execution of an ECMO program can begin. Program leadership must be identified.

Because ECLS is used as a tool to support patients with a variety of disease etiologies, program leadership and structure can also vary widely. Physician leadership should have an extensive knowledge of critical care and mechanical circulatory support. The physician leader(s) work closely with a nursing leader and an administrator to implement, maintain, and oversee the program. Higher-volume centers also require 1 or more full time ECLS coordinators. The ECLS coordinator assists with protocol development, equipment management, and performance data. These roles work together to define the vision of the program.

Outreach and Inreach

As initiation of the ECMO program occurs, program leadership should plan for outreach with regional facilities as well as inreach within the program's own facility. Through the market analysis, regional facilities with patients who are likely to fall within the program's criteria can be identified. It is then important to inform the regional facilities of the program's availability and its patient criteria. The same should be performed with internal groups. Informing all services that could encounter ECLS candidates is crucial to ensuring patients are referred for ECLS at the optimal time.

Financial Assessment and Business Plan

Initiation of an ECMO program requires significant infrastructure investment. Capital equipment, disposable equipment, and the potential need for additional staffing result in significant initial costs for the center. Financial modeling based on patient volumes, predicted costs, reimbursement, and future growth can assist in supporting the viability of the program.

Identifying a partner within the medical coding department to identify appropriate charge description masters is important to capture appropriate ECLS charges. Working with information technology to leverage the electronic medical records to support ECLS documentation also ensures appropriate charge capture. Continual evaluation and oversight of charge capture is important to maximize the program's financial contribution the heath care center as a whole. Once the ECMO program is active, reoccurring periodic review with partners regarding coding, charge capture, and finance ensure program and hospital leadership are aware of the financial impact of the program on the institution as a whole.

TECHNOLOGY AND EQUIPMENT

The advancement of ECLS technology in recent years has allowed for the miniaturization of fully equipped consoles with the capability of providing full or partial cardiopulmonary support outside of the OR theater.[2,3] Unfortunately, this new technology involves a significant financial commitment that must be factored into the initial program development plans. The program director, ECMO coordinator, and clinical perfusionists should collaborate in the initial stage to evaluate all potential clinical considerations and modalities in which the institution desires to use ECMO support. All proposed equipment expenditures need to be presented and reviewed by individual centers' own formulary committee. Staffing models and training should also be discussed in the initial strategic planning prior to equipment purchases. All efforts should be taken to ensure uniformity of devices and equipment, which provides a cost-effective pathway to ensure high levels of patient safety, consistency in functionality, and proficiency for all clinical staff. It is imperative that a clinical perfusionist be included in the equipment decision process to ensure adequate clinical needs are addressed. Perfusionists are specifically trained in extracorporeal circulatory support and can offer valuable feedback.

There are various options available for ECLS consoles and disposable products on the market. The essential equipment consists of a centrifugal blood pump, flow meter, membrane oxygenator, circuit tubing, and oxygen flow regulator along with a method to monitor in vitro pressures and saturations in the ECMO circuitry. Temperature regulation is also often needed; therefore, a circulating water bath heating unit must be readily available. All components should be conveniently kept on an equipment cart for easy deployment.

Pumps

When assessing the needs of a developing an ECMO program, pump selection is a key component for strategic planning. The need for a durable, safe device with adequate backup emergency power and mobility capabilities is paramount in today's workplace. Centrifugal ECLS pumps have proved reliable in supporting all patient demographics in the ECMO population. Important safety mechanisms have recently been integrated into the software to assist in patient and device monitoring. The Cardiohelp system (Maquet, Wayne, New Jersey) provides instant pressure and saturation monitoring, bubble detection, and intervention capabilities conveniently packaged into 1 portable console that can be deployed within or outside the hospital setting. Other centrifugal consoles have proved reliable (ie, Bio-Medicus [Medtronic, Eden Prairie, Minnesota] and CentriMag [Thoratec, Pleasanton, California] pumps); however, most require the purchasing of various external components to monitor circuit pressures and saturations. These additional expenses should be considered in the planning stages of program development.

Heater/Cooler

Temperature control management in ECMO is a requirement. The purchase of heater coolers for each complete ECMO system should be required. It is important to regulate a patient's temperature during ECLS; moderate temperature loss via the ECLS circuitry should be expected because blood is exposed to large surface areas out of the body while circulating. Also, targeted temperature control is now recommended in international resuscitation guidelines; therefore, controlled hypothermia is often implemented in cases of acute cardiac arrest to provide neuroprotection.

Monitors

Appropriate monitoring of the patient and circuit during ECMO support is key to successful clinical outcomes. In-line blood gas monitoring and mixed venous saturation along with hemoglobin/hematocrit values provide essential data related to circuit function and can alert clinical personnel when abnormal conditions are presented during ECLS therapy. Several models are available for ICU use. The CDI System 500 extracorporeal in-line blood gas monitor (Terumo Cardiovascular Group [Ann Arbor, Michigan]) has proved a reliable tool for ECLS monitoring. New advancements in console development may someday include many of these capabilities.

Blood Analyzers

Acquiring point-of-care analyzers can be an important component in patient care management of the ECLS patient. ECMO support presents the unique challenge of inhibiting coagulation within the extracorporeal circuit while avoiding patient-related bleeding or thrombosis complications. Many investigators have described periods off heparin while addressing long-term support or bleeding complications. The interplay between anticoagulation, thrombosis, and bleeding is beyond the scope of this article. All ECMO programs should have hematologists/coagulation experts who contribute to the ECMO team, and some round on patients daily. Unfractionated heparin infusion continues to be the standard for achieving therapeutic anticoagulation. Blood gas analysis and coagulation monitoring are vital tools that ECMO specialists and practitioners can use to rapidly assess and possibly intervene during the ECLS course prior to an adverse occurrence. Laboratory specialists can assist in the initial training and competency requirements needed to comply with laboratory regulations.

Disposables

Basic ECMO circuitry requires conduit tubing packs that can be specifically designed to an individual centers request or standard issued packs supplied by industry vendors. During the program development phase, all participating surgical participants should collaborate to have consensus on what the circuit specifications should look like for all patient demographics and interdepartmental uses. Cannula brands and sizes should be discussed in great detail to avoid excess expenditures and multiple versions of in-house inventory stocked and maintained. Standardization of supplies and equipment enhances team awareness of the ECLS circuit, thus allowing proficiency in an expedient manner. Recent studies have also correlated standardization of medical equipment with substantially reduced risk for errors.

Membrane Oxygenators

Commercial gas exchange devices have improved in recent years. Functionality and reliability are no longer obstacles to extended support duration. Membrane oxygenators can be purchased separately for ECLS systems with uncoupled components (Rotaflow [Maquet]) or purchased in all-inclusive tubing packs (Cardiohelp). Many programs attempt to standardize equipment between the OR perfusion team and the ECMO program.

Cannula

Various catheters are available for commercial use throughout the cardiovascular industry. Cannulas for venoarterial (VA) and venovenous (VV) modalities are necessary to match the access to the ECMO technique. Recently, ambulatory ECMO is recommended as preferable during bridge to lung transplant. Many institutions are using ambulatory VV ECMO for adult respiratory support and in hybrid form (VA/VV) to allow bridge from cardiopulmonary resuscitation to gas exchange support only. Both open and percutaneous cannulation techniques have been described for neonates, children, and adults for cardiopulmonary resuscitation, cardiac support, and total/partial gas exchange. Various sizes of cannulas should be readily available to meet patient-specific requirements, programmatic needs, and physician capability.

Facility Planning

ECLS patients should be located within designated areas within the facility based on the patient population served. Depending on the anticipated patient volume, this could be within 1 or more ICUs. When determining this location it is important to consider physician coverage, staff education and experience, and the potential effect on throughput. ECLS centers with anticipated low volumes should cohort all ECLS patients within 1 ICU. This maximizes the benefit from ECLS education and experience for both physicians and staff.

Just as a determining the location of ECLS patients is important, so is the location of ECLS equipment and supplies. Ideally, these items are kept in 1 location as well.

Location should be determined based on the highest volume cannulation location. Typically, equipment and supplies are located near ORs, catheterization laboratories, and/or ICUs. Because the equipment and supplies represent a significant investment from the facility, the location should be secure but also easily accessed by designated staff. During the time there is a patient on ECLS, a protocol must be in place for ready access to back-up equipment. In the instance of equipment failure, staff must be aware of the back-up location and personnel must be assigned to obtain back up equipment.

TEAM BUILDING/STAFF MODELS

In the initial stages of program development, a core group of providers and staff should be identified as those who cannulate, manage, and provide care to ECLS patients.[2,4,5] To support these highly complex patients, a center must have a multidisciplinary team comprised of many specialized disciplines. At a minimum, an ECMO program requires collaboration from cardiothoracic surgery, cardiology, anesthesiology, intensivists, perfusion, nursing, radiology, palliative medicine, respiratory therapy, physical and occupation therapy, pharmacy, clinical laboratory, blood bank, and biomedical engineering. These patients frequently require additional consults from neurology, nephrology, pediatrics, and infectious disease. During the planning stages, an evaluation of these services and each area's capability to support an ECMO program should be assessed. Additional staffing needs should be identified and addressed at this stage in planning.

At this time, program and hospital leadership should outline the requirements for cannulation privileges. Leadership should also outline the process for patient identification and the decision making for proceeding with ECLS. Many ECLS centers require input for 2 providers prior to ECLS initiation. This ensures appropriate patient selection and can decrease the occurrence of futile ECLS cases.

Staffing models for daily management of ECLS patients vary widely among centers. Delineation of role responsibilities should be assigned for ECLS initiation, daily circuit evaluation and maintenance, ECLS complications, and ECLS discontinuations. Despite the patient management model, all programs typically involve physicians, advanced practice providers, nursing staff, perfusion, and ECLS specialists. It is important to involve members from each of these disciplines in program development, training, and quality assurance to build and maintain a cohesive and successful ECLS program. Multiple staffing models have been described, but ultimately ECMO personnel must be accountable to the ECMO protocols.

Guidelines for Training and Continuous Education of Extracorporeal Membrane Oxygenation Specialists

The development of training guidelines for all involved disciplines participating in the management of ECLS patients should be established in the initial planning of a new ECMO program. The ELSO has established comprehensive recommended guidelines that provide a clinical foundation for the support of ECLS therapy. Training recommendations are outlined.

Initial training

1. Didactic course: 24 hours to 36 hours of didactic lectures focusing on the following topics:
   - Introduction to ECMO therapy
   - Physiology of diseases treated with ECMO

- Criteria and contraindication for ECMO
- Pre-EMCO procedures
- Physiology of coagulation
- ECMO equipment
- Physiology of VA and VV ECMO
- Daily patient and circuit management on ECMO
- Emergencies and complication during ECMO
- Management of complex ECMO cases
- Weaning from ECMO (techniques and complications)
- Decannulation techniques
- Post-ECMO complications
- Ethical and social issues
- Short-term and long-term outcomes of ECMO patients

2. Water drills: 16 hours to 32 hours
   - Hands-on wet laboratories designed to familiarize practitioners with ECMO circuitry and components, cannulas, and membrane oxygenators
   - Emergency management procedures
3. Animal/simulation laboratories: 24 hours to 72 hours
   Small group sessions designed to simulate daily ECMO management
   - Blood gas access and sampling
   - Blood gas analysis and management
   - Flowsheet documentation
   - Protocol/guideline management
   - Emergency intervention techniques
4. Competency testing: written and/or oral examination
   ECMO coordinator and ECMO director establish center standards.

Continuing education
Continuing education planning must be developed and budgeted for in the initial planning phase for new ECMO programs. Continuing education opportunities should be developed inside the facility for ECMO specialists and participating advanced practitioners. In addition, annual regional or national meeting attendance should be made available to ECMO staff.

ICU nursing education should be established with the support of staff development. All disciplines that are expected to have regular contact with ECLS patients should have a basic understanding of the principles of ECLS therapy. Disciplines that should receive basic awareness training are

- CT intensive care nursing
- Advanced practice registered nursing
- Pharmacy
- Physical and occupational therapy

Policies and Protocols

- Clinical practice guidelines are essential for comprehensive standards established by each ECMO center. The ELSO provides general guidelines that can be used for basic recommendations for ECMO management[2]; however, center-specific protocols and guidelines should be drafted with the input of a multidisciplinary team consisting of practitioners who provide joint daily management of ECLS patients. The development of specific procedural guidelines can mitigate intrinsic risk associated with ECLS therapy and allow for clinical consistency and quality assurance throughout a patient's ECLS course. Quality improvement initiatives can easily be identified and addressed when a central starting point has been established.

- When considering the implementation of an ECMO program, a comprehensive inclusion and exclusion criteria should be drafted to establish parameters in which ECLS therapy is offered. Reports have shown that initial selection process directly correlates with positive clinical outcomes. Clear criteria for the initiation of ECMO should include guidelines, such as treatment of severe cardiac or respiratory failure that is unresponsive to conventional management. General guidelines for daily management, such as sedation, anticoagulation, and ventilator management, should be collectively agreed on among the core practitioners. A detailed process for weaning and trialing off VA support or VV support should also be established. Communication with supporting elements, such as respiratory, radiology, and echography departments, should also be established to define their role and process for providing services to ECLS patients.

Program Evaluation

- A formal process for quality assurance and improvement must be established when developing a new ECMO program. The ELSO guidelines recommend routine internal program reviews to assess clinical performance and overall outcomes. The ECMO director with assistance from the ECMO coordinator should develop a pathway to routinely review program essentials. The hospital chief medical officer should be involved in this stage of planning.
- Quarterly meetings with the entire ECMO clinical management team should be held to discuss an administrative overview of the program. These meetings should consist of topics that address program development and operational needs along with equipment and financial reviews. Quarterly morbidity and mortality reviews should be incorporated into the program standards. Multidisciplinary case reviews should be conducted after every ECLS run to ensure process development, quality assurance, and valued care are always at the forefront.
- Data collection and a formal process to report an ECMO program's viability to hospital administration should be established in the initial development of a new program. The ECMO director should identify a central process and a point person to oversee that proper collection and reporting of data are consistent.
- The ELSO provides an international registry that voluntarily collects centers' individual reported data and offers clinical research support, quality assessment, and regulatory updates related to ECMO therapy.[6] The ELSO consortium consists of physicians, nurses, perfusionists, respiratory therapists, and clinical researchers from various health care institutions dedicated to the advancement of ECMO therapy. Clinical benchmarking can be assessed and tracked with the use of ELSO registry data. Biannual and annual US and international summary reports are released for open review of current ECMO outcomes, modalities, and initial diagnostic indications. Institutional membership participation should be pursued by any new developing center to provide guidance for future and ongoing program assessment and evaluation. Membership in the ELSO is highly recommended.

REFERENCES

1. Sauer CM, Yuh DD, Bonde P. Extracorporeal membrane oxygenation use has increased by 433% in adults in the United States from 2006 to 2011. ASAIO J 2015;61:31–6.

2. Extracorporeal Life Support Organization. ELSO guidelines for ECMO centers, Version 1.8. 2014. Available at: https://www.elso.org/portals/0/igd/archive/filemanager/faf3f6a3c7cusersshyerdocumentselsoguidelinesecmocentersv1.8.pdf. Accessed July 2, 2017.
3. Keselman A, Tang X, Patel V, et al. Institutional decision-making for medical device purchasing: evaluating patient safety. Stud Health Technol Inform 2004;107(Pt 2): 1357–61.
4. Annich GM, Lynch WB, MacLaren G, et al, editors. ECMO extracorporeal cardio-pulmonary support in critical care. 4th edition. Ann Arbor (MI): Extracorporeal Life Support Organization; 2012.
5. Short BL, Williams L, editors. ECMO specialist training manual. Ann Arbor (MI): Extracorporeal Life Support Organization; 2010.
6. ECMO Registry of Extracorporeal Life Support Organization. Available at: https://www.elso.org/Registry.aspx. Accessed May 31, 2017.

Cardiac Support
Emphasis on Venoarterial ECMO

Christopher S. King, MD[a],*, Aviral Roy, MBBS[b], Liam Ryan, MD[c],
Ramesh Singh, MD[c]

KEYWORDS

- Venoarterial extracorporeal membrane support • Cardiogenic shock
- Extracorporeal cardiopulmonary resuscitation • Pulmonary hypertension
- Pulmonary embolism

KEY POINTS

- Venoarterial extracorporeal membrane oxygenation (ECMO) can be used as a bridge to recovery or definitive therapy for several conditions, including cardiogenic shock, pulmonary embolism, intoxication or poisoning, and hypothermia.
- Important considerations when developing a cannulation strategy for venoarterial ECMO include cardiac and pulmonary function, need for mobilization, anticipated duration of support, and the urgency of the time to cannulation.
- Careful management of patients having venoarterial ECMO is required to minimize the risk of common complications, including limb ischemia, bleeding, infection, thrombosis, and cerebral ischemia.

INTRODUCTION

In 1972, the first successful use of venoarterial (VA) extracorporeal membrane oxygenation (ECMO) was reported in a 24-year old man who was severely injured in a motorcycle accident.[1] After 3 days, the patient was weaned from ECMO and eventually recovered. Major advances in extracorporeal support have been made since this groundbreaking first case. Increasing experience, as well as advances in ECMO equipment and options for definitive therapy following ECMO support, have led to improved outcomes and increased use of this technology.[2] Since data collection started in 1990, support of more than 10,000 adult patients with VA ECMO has been reported to the Extracorporeal Life Support Organization (ELSO) registry, with 40% of these patients surviving to hospital discharge.[3] This article provides an

Conflicts of Interest: The authors have no conflicts to disclose.
[a] Department of Medicine, Inova Fairfax Hospital, 3300 Gallows Road, Falls Church, VA 22042, USA; [b] Department of Critical Care, Cooper University Hospital, 427C Dorrance, 1 Cooper Plaza, Camden, NJ 08103, USA; [c] Department of Cardiothoracic Surgery, Inova Fairfax Hospital, 3300 Gallows Road, Falls Church, VA 22042, USA
* Corresponding author. 18674 Fawn Ridge Lane, Reston, VA 20194.
E-mail address: Christopher.king@inova.org

Crit Care Clin 33 (2017) 777–794
http://dx.doi.org/10.1016/j.ccc.2017.06.002
0749-0704/17/© 2017 Elsevier Inc. All rights reserved.

overview of VA ECMO for clinicians not well versed in this technology. It first discusses the components of the VA ECMO circuit and contrasts VA ECMO with venovenous (VV) ECMO. It then addresses patient selection, including indications and contraindications to use of ECMO. It next covers cannulation strategies and basic management of VA ECMO, including commonly encountered complications.

WHAT IS VENOARTERIAL EXTRACORPOREAL MEMBRANE OXYGENATION AND HOW DOES IT DIFFER FROM VENOVENOUS EXTRACORPOREAL MEMBRANE OXYGENATION?

The basic components of any ECMO circuit include a cannula to drain blood from the venous system (inflow cannula), a pump, an oxygenator, and a cannula to return blood to the body (outflow cannula). In addition to these essential components, most ECMO circuits contain a console where pump speed can be adjusted, a heat exchanger, various ports for blood sampling and medication infusion, a saturation sensor on the inflow cannula, and a flow sensor on the outflow cannula. The inflow cannula generally sits in the right atrium or inferior vena cava (IVC). Modern adult ECMO circuits are typically powered by a centrifugal pump, which rapidly rotates a magnetically levitated impeller, generating negative pressure and entraining blood into the circuit. The entrained venous blood is then passed through a membrane oxygenator, which facilitates gas exchange. In the oxygenator, blood separated by a porous membrane is passed by a countercurrent sweep gas, allowing oxygen to enter the blood, carbon dioxide to be removed, and heat to be exchanged[4] (**Fig. 1**). The now oxygenated and warmed blood is delivered through the outflow cannula to the body. More detailed explanation of the individual circuit components is beyond the scope of this article but can be found elsewhere.[4,5]

In VV ECMO, the superoxygenated blood in the outflow cannula is delivered to the venous system, where it then traverses the pulmonary circulation and is pumped to the body by the native left ventricular (LV) output. This system allows respiratory support in patients with impaired gas exchange by bolstering the oxygen content of blood delivered to the right side of the heart. VV ECMO provides no direct hemodynamic support, although hemodynamic benefit is often seen with the initiation of VV ECMO because hypoxia, hypercarbia, and acidosis improve

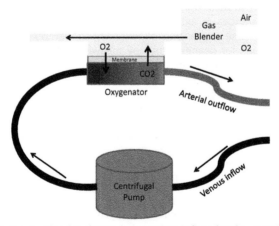

Fig. 1. An ECMO circuit. Blood is drawn into venous inflow by the centrifugal pump. It is then pumped through an oxygenator where the blood is separated from a countercurrent gas flow by a thin permeable membrane. Oxygen enters the blood and carbon dioxide is removed. The oxygenated and decarboxylated blood is then returned to the body.

and the adverse cardiac effects of high-level ventilator support required for respiratory failure are mitigated. In VA ECMO, the outflow cannula bypasses the heart and lungs and delivers oxygenated blood with a pressure that provide both respiratory and hemodynamic support. By doing so, VA ECMO not only augments the native cardiac output with returned flow but also unloads the failing heart by decreasing preload.[6] **Table 1** provides a comparison of the hemodynamic effects of VV and VA ECMO.

VA ECMO can provide 60% to 80% of predicted resting cardiac output.[7] Targeted flow rates in adults are generally 60 to 80 mL/kg/min.[8] ECMO flow rates are affected by preload, afterload, and the revolutions per minute (RPM) of the centrifugal pump. Preload delivery to the pump depends on the length and diameter of the inflow cannulas as well as patient volume status. Circuits are also afterload sensitive. Kinking of the outflow cannula, thrombus in the oxygenator, or high systemic vascular resistance can all decrease ECMO flow rates. These issues are discussed in greater detail later in this article.

HOW TO SELECT APPROPRIATE PATIENTS FOR VENOARTERIAL EXTRACORPOREAL MEMBRANE OXYGENATION. WHAT ARE THE INDICATIONS AND CONTRAINDICATIONS?
General Considerations

Initiation of extracorporeal support is a complex, resource-intensive undertaking that requires careful consideration and should only be performed at centers with sufficient resources to care for this patient population. Appropriate patient selection is of paramount importance. Given the lack of robust data supporting its efficacy, the cost, and the potential for complications, ECMO support should only be initiated in those patients with an appropriate indication who cannot be managed with more traditional therapies. Clinicians must also remember that ECMO is not a therapy but is a means of bridging to an ultimate destination. For some patients, that destination will be a durable ventricular assist device (VAD) or cardiac or lung transplant. For others, ECMO will support end-organ perfusion until the initial insult resolves, acting as a bridge to recovery. In some instances, ECMO provides a bridge to decision, providing time to determine whether an insult is recoverable or whether the patient is an appropriate candidate for destination therapies. In summary, before initiation of ECMO support, it is mandatory to ensure that the indication is appropriate and that conventional therapies are inadequate, to consider any contraindications, and to clearly delineate the

Table 1
Hemodynamic effects of venovenous and venoarterial extracorporeal membrane oxygenation

	VA ECMO	VV ECMO
Indication	Cardiac or cardiopulmonary failure	Pulmonary failure
Effect on RV	Decreased preload Decreased afterload	None
Effect on LV	Decreased preload Increased afterload	None
Hemodynamic support	Partial to complete	No direct support; decrease in ventilator support facilitated by VV ECMO may lead to hemodynamic improvement

Abbreviation: RV, right ventricle.

long-term goal of instituting ECMO therapy. **Fig. 2** provides an algorithm for candidate selection for VA ECMO.

Indications for Venoarterial Extracorporeal Membrane Oxygenation

Refractory cardiogenic shock or failure to wean from cardiopulmonary bypass have been the traditional indications for VA ECMO support. Although these indications still account for most VA ECMO use, the technology is being successfully applied to an expanding number of applications (**Table 2**). The major indications for use of VA ECMO are reviewed later, along with outcomes data for each where available.

Refractory Cardiogenic Shock

There are several causes of cardiogenic shock, including myocardial infarction, acute valvular disorders, myocarditis, postpartum cardiomyopathy, takotsubo cardiomyopathy, postcardiotomy syndrome, decompensated chronic cardiomyopathy, refractory ventricular arrhythmia, and primary graft failure following heart transplant. Traditional therapy for cardiogenic shock focuses on correcting the underlying cause, optimization of volume status, and use of inotropes and vasopressors to maintain adequate tissue perfusion. The timing of initiation of ECMO for cardiogenic shock is controversial given the paucity of data and lack of guideline recommendations. In general, VA ECMO is initiated in appropriate candidates if there is evidence of ongoing tissue hypoperfusion and worsening end-organ dysfunction in the presence of escalating inotropic and vasopressor support. Outcomes of patients with cardiogenic shock supported with ECMO are poorly delineated because they are based primarily on the reports of case series and vary widely based on the causative condition.[9] Acute myocarditis seems to have the most favorable outcomes, with survival to discharge nearing 70%.[10] A meta-analysis of 4 cohort studies examining outcomes of patients with cardiogenic shock caused by myocardial infarction reported 30-day survival of 55% for those treated with VA ECMO compared with 29.7% for those treated with intra-aortic balloon pump.[11] Outcomes for postcardiotomy syndrome, defined as the inability to wean from cardiopulmonary bypass or need for mechanical support

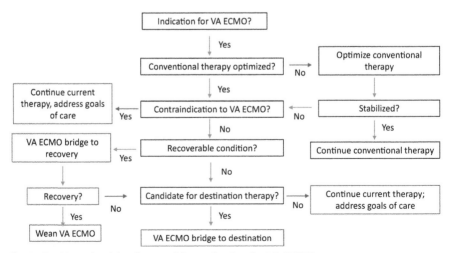

Fig. 2. Decision algorithm for candidate selection for VA ECMO.

Table 2
Indications and contraindications to venoarterial extracorporeal membrane oxygenation

Indications for VA ECMO	Contraindications to VA ECMO
Refractory cardiogenic shock	Absolute contraindications
• Acute coronary syndrome	• Aortic dissection
• Myocarditis	• Severe aortic regurgitation
• Peripartum cardiomyopathy	• End-stage cardiac dysfunction without
• Decompensated cardiomyopathy	destination (VAD or transplant)
• Primary graft failure after heart transplant	• End-stage pulmonary dysfunction in non–
Postcardiotomy shock	transplant candidate
Recurrent life-threatening arrhythmia	• Irreversible, severe neurologic injury
ECPR	Relative contraindication
Massive pulmonary embolism	• Advanced age
Accidental hypothermia	• Hepatic failure
Drug overdose	• Advanced malignancy
Poisoning	• Active bleeding
Periprocedural circulatory support for high	• Contraindication to anticoagulation (eg
risk procedures	intracranial hemorrhage)
Septic shock	
Air embolism	
Anaphylactic shock	
Traumatic injury to the heart or great vessels	
Pulmonary hypertension	
Facilitation of transfer of critically ill patients	

Abbreviation: ECPR, extracorporeal cardiopulmonary resuscitation.

in the immediate postoperative period following cardiac surgery, are poor, with most studies reporting rates of survival to hospital discharge of 25% to 50%.[12]

Predicting survival in individual patients before initiating VA ECMO is difficult. Data extracted from the ELSO registry on 3846 patients treated with VA ECMO were used to develop a clinical prediction tool (www.save-score.com) to estimate survival of patients with cardiogenic shock.[13] It should be noted that patients treated with extracorporeal cardiopulmonary resuscitation (ECPR) were excluded from this cohort so the tool cannot be extrapolated to this population.

Extracorporeal Cardiopulmonary Resuscitation

Survival of both in-hospital cardiac arrest (IHCA) and out-of-hospital cardiac arrest (OHCA) treated with conventional cardiopulmonary resuscitation (CCPR) is low, estimated at 15% to 20% and 10%, respectively.[14] ECPR refers to the rapid initiation of VA ECMO support in the context of refractory cardiac arrest. ECPR has been used in patients with IHCA in the cardiac catheterization laboratory or on the ward and in patients presenting to the emergency department with OHCA. It is hypothesized that use of ECPR can restore perfusion more rapidly and, in turn, improve both survival and neurologic outcomes. To date, CCPR and ECPR have not been compared in a randomized, controlled trial. A recent meta-analysis of 6 trials (3 IHCA, 2 OHCA, 1 mixed) containing 2260 patients concluded that ECPR improved both survival and long-term neurologic outcome. Survival rates in the ECPR arms ranged from 14.5% to 34.9% compared with 6.4% to 21.7% in the CCPR arm.[15] Criteria regarding candidacy for ECPR following cardiac arrest are a matter of debate. In general, patients must have had a witnessed arrest, minimal interruptions to cardiopulmonary resuscitation, presumed cardiac origin or pulmonary embolism (PE) as the cause of the arrest, and be less than 75 years of age.[16]

Massive Pulmonary Embolism

Massive PE can cause acute right ventricular failure resulting in cardiogenic shock or cardiac arrest, and is associated with a high mortality. Conventional treatment includes systemic or catheter-directed thrombolysis or surgical embolectomy. VA ECMO can provide cardiopulmonary support for PE while allowing the clot to resolve with anticoagulation alone or may serve a bridge to a surgical or catheter-directed therapy. **Box 1** details various uses of VA ECMO in the treatment of massive PE.

In 2015, Yusuff and colleagues[17] published a review of the reported cases of PE managed with VA ECMO to date. A total of 78 patients (11 case reports and 8 case series) were reported on, 43 (55%) of whom had a cardiac arrest. Overall survival of the cohort was 70.1%. For patients who presented with cardiac arrest there was a survival of 49%, compared with a historical rate as high as 75%. Based on the available data, use of VA ECMO may be a reasonable management strategy for a select group of patients with massive PE, including patients with clot in transit, marked hemodynamic instability at high risk for cardiac arrest, or unstable patients presenting to facilities with inability to provide definitive therapy for massive PE.

Accidental Hypothermia

Excellent outcomes have been seen with the use of VA ECMO for rewarming of patients with cardiac arrest secondary to hypothermia, with rates of survival and good neurologic outcome of 67.7% and 61.5% respectively.[18] It should be highlighted that these results only apply to patients with cardiac arrest primarily caused by cold exposure and not with primary hypoxic arrest with associated hypothermia (eg, drowning, avalanche).[18]

Septic Shock

The use of VA ECMO for refractory septic shock remains controversial. Survival to hospital discharge reported in 3 recent cohort studies was a dismal 15% to 30%.[19–21] In contrast, a case series of VA ECMO therapy for septic shock complicated by severe LV dysfunction published by Brechot and colleagues[22] reported an impressive survival rate of 70%. One major reason for these discordant findings is that

---

Box 1
Clinical strategies for venoarterial extracorporeal membrane oxygenation in acute massive pulmonary embolism

Marked hemodynamic instability
- Bridge to recovery
- Bridge to embolectomy
- Bridge to catheter-directed thrombolysis
- Bridge to percutaneous thrombus removal

Hemodynamic instability with contraindication to systemic thrombolysis
- Bridge to recovery
- Bridge to catheter-directed thrombolysis

Clot in transit
- Bridge to embolectomy
- Bridge to percutaneous thrombus removal

Escalation of care
- Transfer to referral center for definitive therapy

ECPR after massive PE and cardiac arrest

Brechot and colleagues[19–22] initiated VA ECMO early (mean of 24 hours) and before arrest in all patients in their cohort, whereas the other series included patients who had cardiac arrest. Limited success with early initiation of VA ECMO in patients with septic shock with cardiac dysfunction has been achieved, but further research is required.

Pulmonary Hypertension

VA ECMO can serve as a bridge to recovery or lung transplant in patients with decompensated pulmonary hypertension. In patients with a reversible insult, ECMO can provide support while pulmonary vasodilator therapy and volume status are optimized. In those with end-stage pulmonary hypertension, ECMO can provide a bridge to lung transplant. Several innovative cannulation strategies have been used to provide ECMO support in patients with pulmonary hypertension, including (1) internal jugular venous drainage with subclavian arterial return, (2) drainage from the main pulmonary artery with reinfusion into the left atrium via sternotomy, and (3) use of a VV ECMO dual-lumen bicaval cannula to withdraw from the IVC with the reinfusion jet directed at an atrial septal defect or patent foramen ovale creating an oxygenated right-to-left shunt.[23]

Additional Indications

Other instances in which VA ECMO support has been successfully applied include poisoning or overdose, anaphylaxis, traumatic injury to the heart or great vessels, and for periprocedural support for high-risk cardiac interventions.[24–27] In addition, VA ECMO support has been used to stabilize critically ill patients for transport to tertiary care centers offering therapies unavailable at the referring center.[28]

Contraindications to Venoarterial Extracorporeal Membrane Oxygenation

Very few absolute contraindications to VA ECMO exist. There is general consensus that initiation of ECMO support in patients with irreversible major organ dysfunction without a means to correct it (eg, transplant, VAD) is inappropriate. Severe aortic insufficiency precludes VA ECMO use, because the return flow to the aorta would result in severe LV distention and pulmonary edema. Several relative contraindications exist, including advanced age, incurable malignancy, uncontrolled bleeding or other contraindication to anticoagulation, and morbid obesity. **Table 2** lists absolute and relative contraindications to ECMO.

THE DECISION HAS BEEN MADE TO PROCEED WITH EXTRACORPOREAL MEMBRANE OXYGENATION. HOW IS THE OPTIMAL CANNULATION STRATEGY DETERMINED?

Once the decision to initiate VA ECMO is made, the cannulation strategy must be determined. Several factors must be considered when determining the optimal cannulation strategy, including the urgency of the situation, the underlying cardiac issue (right, left, or biventricular heart failure), pulmonary status, the size of arterial vessels, the need for mobilization, and the anticipated duration of support. Consideration must also be given to the size of the cannulas to ensure that flows adequate to provide full support can be achieved. Cannulation can be performed centrally, through a sternotomy or thoracotomy, or peripherally.

Central Cannulation

Because of the need for thoracotomy or sternotomy, central cannulation is most commonly encountered in patients who are unable to wean from cardiopulmonary bypass. In this scenario, the cannula used for intraoperative cardiopulmonary bypass can be connected to the VA ECMO circuit. The inflow cannula typically drains the right atrium, whereas the outflow cannula instills blood into the ascending aorta.[7] Central cannulation is also sometimes used as an alternative to cardiopulmonary bypass during lung transplant.[29] Advantages of central cannulation include adequate delivery of oxygenated blood to the upper body and the ability to deliver high flow rates given the large cannula diameters. Disadvantages of central cannulation include the need for operative placement and removal, limited ability to mobilize the patient, and increased bleeding and infection risk.[30]

Peripheral Cannulation

Peripheral cannulation is performed either percutaneously or by vascular cutdown. Percutaneous placement is performed via the Seldinger technique. Ultrasonography evaluation is useful in both accessing the vessels and in evaluating the size of vessels before cannulation. Thrombus, vascular stenosis, peripheral arterial disease, and prior vascular surgical procedures may render percutaneous cannulation difficult or impossible in some cases.[31] Advantages of percutaneous cannulation include decreased bleeding and infection risk, potential for patient mobilization, ability to cannulate at the bedside, and ability to cannulate expediently. Disadvantages of peripheral cannulation include vascular compromise of extremities, upper body hypoxemia, and development of aortic root or intracardiac thrombus (caused by LV distention caused by increased afterload from the ECMO return flow in patients with minimal LV contractility).[32]

Venous (Inflow) Cannula

The inflow cannula drains blood from the right atrium via the right internal jugular vein, subclavian vein, or the femoral vein. Venous cannulas of the greatest diameter and shortest length possible should be used to optimize preload to the circuit. Larger patients may require a second inflow cannula if adequate drainage cannot be achieved with a single inflow cannula.[7] Venous cannula are typically 19 to 25 Fr.[32] Both end and side holes are generally present on venous cannulas to facilitate drainage if the end of the cannula becomes occluded.

Arterial (Outflow) Cannula

Multiple sites can be used for the returned of oxygenated blood to the proximal arterial system. The femoral artery is a commonly used location for the outflow cannula when providing VA ECMO support. This vessel can be accessed percutaneously or by cutdown. The cannula should terminate in the common iliac artery or abdominal aorta. Complications of femoral arterial cannulation include limb ischemia, LV distention and pulmonary congestion, and upper body hypoxemia. Limb ischemia can be avoided by placing a perfusion cannula distal to the cannulation site in the femoral artery. This cannula is then perfused with oxygenated blood from a side port off the arterial cannula.[33] The right or left subclavian or axillary arteries can be used for arterial cannulation as well, which requires surgical placement of an end-to-side Dacron graft. These upper extremity arterial cannulation sites have the advantage of decreasing the risk of aortic root thrombosis and upper body hypoxemia. Upper extremity cannulation also may facilitate patient mobilization. Biscotti and Bacchetta[34] of Columbia University Medical Center described a cannulation strategy designed to optimize patient mobilizations using right internal jugular venous drainage and right subclavian arterial return, which they dubbed the Sport Model in 2014.[34] Cannula site hematoma and ipsilateral limb swelling can complicate use of this technique.[34] Although the right common carotid artery is frequently used for VA ECMO cannulation in the pediatric population, it is associated with an increased risk of stroke and not commonly used for adult VA ECMO support.

Arterial cannulas are typically 15 to 25 Fr and of a shorter length than venous cannulas. A recent study by Takayama and colleagues[35] found that smaller 15-Fr cannulas were able to provide support comparable with larger 17-Fr to 24-Fr cannulas and caused fewer bleeding complications. No side ports are present on arterial cannulas because they result in turbulent blood flow. The appropriate site for monitoring of arterial blood gases in patients on VA ECMO varies with the location of the arterial cannula. For instance, a right subclavian arterial cannula directs flow down the right arm, resulting in falsely increased blood oxygen levels in samples drawn from a right radial arterial line. It is therefore recommended that arterial blood samples in these patients be drawn from a left radial arterial line. **Table 3** lists the potential advantages and complications of the various arterial cannulation locations and the recommended site for arterial blood gas monitoring of each.

TRIPLE CANNULATION STRATEGIES
Venoarteriovenous Extracorporeal Membrane Oxygenation

As briefly mentioned earlier, upper body hypoxemia can complicate the care of patients who are peripherally cannulated for VA ECMO, particularly those with femoral

Table 3
Arterial cannulation locations

Location	Advantages	Disadvantages/ Possible Complications	Recommended Site for ABG Monitoring
Femoral	• Rapid cannulation	• Upper body hypoxemia • LV distention • Limb ischemia	Right radial
Right axillary	• Facilitates mobilization • Lower risk for upper body hypoxia	• Hematoma • Limb swelling • Requires surgical anastomosis	Left radial
Left axillary	• Facilitates mobilization • Lower risk for upper body hypoxia	• Hematoma • Limb swelling • Requires surgical anastomosis	Right radial
Central cannulation (ascending aorta)	• High flows possible • No upper body hypoxemia	• Bleeding risk increased • Infection risk increased • Requires sternotomy or thoracotomy • Requires surgery for decannulation	Right or left radial
Right common carotid	• Facilitates mobilization • Lower risk for upper body hypoxia	• Increased risk of stroke	Left radial

Abbreviation: ABG, arterial blood gas.

arterial cannulas. If a patient recovers ventricular function while still experiencing significant pulmonary dysfunction, the native cardiac output will pump poorly oxygenated blood to the coronary arteries and brain while well-oxygenated blood from the ECMO outflow cannula only reaches the lower half of the body. This phenomenon is known as north-south syndrome, harlequin syndrome, or differential cyanosis and may lead to coronary or cerebral ischemia. One strategy to overcome this is to split the arterial outflow with a Y connector and deliver highly oxygenated blood to the right internal jugular vein. This technique increases the oxygen content delivered through the pulmonary circulation to the left ventricle, improving oxygen delivery to the brain and heart. The relative flows of the 2 outflow cannulas can be modulated by clamps and should be monitored carefully.[32] This cannulation configuration is commonly referred to as venoarteriovenous ECMO.[7] Additional ways to combat differential cyanosis are summarized in **Table 4**.

Venovenoarterial Extracorporeal Membrane Oxygenation

Venovenoarterial ECMO refers to the addition of a second venous drainage cannula, usually to the right internal jugular vein, in patients with a preexisting femoral venous inflow and femoral arterial outflow cannulas. The 2 venous cannulas can be joined with a Y connector. This configuration is indicated for patients with marked LV distention caused by inadequate drainage or in patients whose small vessel size precludes placement of a large enough drainage cannula to provide adequate preload to the circuit.[32]

Table 4
Common complications of venoarterial extracorporeal membrane oxygenation

Complication	Possible Sequelae	Possible Management Strategies
Loss of pulsatility	• LV or aortic root thrombosis • LV distention and ischemia • Pulmonary edema or hemorrhage	• Add inotropes • Decrease VA ECMO flow • Intra-aortic balloon pump • Direct LV decompression • Percutaneous LVAD
Upper body hypoxemia or differential cyanosis	• Cerebral ischemia • Coronary ischemia	• Treat pulmonary disorder • Increase ventilator support • Increase VA ECMO flows • Place upper body arterial cannula • Venoarteriovenous configuration
Limb ischemia	• Loss of limb	• Place a distal perfusion catheter • Move femoral cannula to upper body artery (subclavian or axillary)
Bleeding	• Hypotension • Inadequate oxygen delivery • Low ECMO flows • Death	• Local measures (direct pressure) • Decrease anticoagulation intensity • Surgical evaluation/intervention

Abbreviation: LVAD, left ventricular assist device.

Additional Therapies

Several additional options for mechanical support in cardiogenic shock exist. Percutaneously inserted left ventricular assist devices (LVADs), such as the TandemHeart (Cardiac Assist, Inc, Pittsburgh, PA) and Impella (Abiomed) devices, are available to provide temporary LV support.[36] The TandemHeart device can also be configured to provide VV ECMO support.[37] Temporary right ventricle (RV) support can be achieved with the Centrimag (Levitrnix LLC, Waltham, MA) or Impella RP (Abiomed).[38] A detailed discussion of these devices is beyond the scope of this article.

How to Manage Patients Who Are Cannulated and on Extracorporeal Membrane Oxygenation Support

The management of VA ECMO patients is complex. The approach to support should be individualized based on the hemodynamic needs of the patient. Careful monitoring is required to ensure adequacy of support. Vigilance is also required to detect and correct frequently encountered complications in a timely manner. An overview of the basic management and monitoring of VA ECMO is provided here, and commonly encountered complications and the recommended corrective actions are also highlighted (**Table 5**).

Table 5 Troubleshooting guide for commonly encountered monitoring issues	
Issue	Potential Corrective Actions

Low flow	• Inadequate preload
	  ○ Administer volume or transfuse
	  ○ Assess for bleeding
	  ○ Assess for inlet cannula kinking
	• Increased afterload
	  ○ Assess for kinking of outflow cannula
	  ○ Assess for pump thrombus
	  ○ Decrease MAP with antihypertensives
	• Increase RPM

Low MAP	• Assess for bleeding, systemic infection • Administer volume or transfuse • Start vasopressor • Increase ECMO flow
Low Pao_2	• Increase circuit Fio_2 • Increase circuit flow • Assess oxygenator function • Increase ventilator support
Increased Pco_2	• Increase sweep gas flow • Increase ventilator support
Low Svo_2	• Increase ECMO flow • Ensure Pao_2 adequate • Transfuse blood

Increased lactate level	• Assess for local ischemia (gut, limb)
	• Increase systemic O_2 delivery
	  ○ Increase ECMO flow
	  ○ Transfuse
	  ○ Increase Pao_2 if low

Abbreviations: Fio_2, fraction of inspired oxygen; MAP, mean arterial pressure; Svo_2, mixed venous oxygen saturation.

HEMODYNAMIC SUPPORT
Determine the Degree of Support Required

The primary goal of ECMO support is to maintain adequate oxygen delivery to end organs.

Delivery of oxygen depends on cardiac output, the hemoglobin concentration, and arterial oxygen saturation. In ECMO patients, all of these variables can be manipulated to ensure adequate tissue perfusion. Recall that, in ECMO patients, the functional cardiac output is a combination of the native cardiac output and the ECMO flow. The optimal amount of ECMO support varies depending on native cardiac function. Patients with severely depressed native cardiac function frequently require maximal ECMO support. In contrast, patients who primarily have RV failure with relatively intact LV function typically only require partial support. The degree of support provided should be tailored to the pathophysiology of the patient being supported.

Optimize Flow

The flow produced by the ECMO circuit depends on the modifiable variables of preload, afterload, and RPM of the centrifugal pump, as well as the static variable of cannula length and diameter.[7] ECMO circuit flow is controlled by adjusting the RPMs of the centrifugal pump. Increasing RPM results in increased ECMO flow, assuming the system is not limited by preload, afterload, or cannula size. In the setting of a stable RPM, decreased flows can result from inadequate preload or increased afterload. Inadequate preload can result from hypovolemia (from bleeding, distributive shock, overdiuresis) or mechanical obstruction (from cardiac tamponade, tension pneumothorax, abdominal compartment syndrome, or cannula malposition or kinking) and typically manifests as chugging or chattering of the circuit and decreased flows.[7] When encountered, temporarily decreasing the RPMs of the pump and providing volume can correct the problem. The patient and circuit should also be inspected for evidence of bleeding or cannula malposition or kinking.

Afterload on the ECMO circuit is affected by the systemic vascular resistance (SVR) as well as resistance in the circuit distal to the pump. Decreased flows caused by increased afterload may be caused by increased SVR (increased mean arterial pressure [MAP]) or increased resistance in the circuit (kinking of the outflow cannula, clot in the oxygenator membrane). If the increase in afterload is caused by an increased SVR, this can be corrected by reducing the MAP with antihypertensives or decreasing vasopressors or inotropes.

Optimize Mean Arterial Pressure

Maintenance of blood flow alone is insufficient to ensure adequate tissue perfusion. A sufficient MAP is essential to maintain perfusion to vital organs, including the heart, brain, and kidneys.[39] There are numerous causes of hypotension in ECMO patients, including vasodilatory effects of sedatives, hypovolemia from volume depletion or bleeding, and distributive shock from sepsis or postcardiotomy vasoplegia. There is much debate over what the optimal minimal MAP goal should be, and it is likely that it varies among individual patients.[40] A reasonable MAP goal for most ECMO patients is 65 to 90 mm Hg. This range allows adequate end-organ perfusion without causing excessive afterload.

MAP is a product of SVR and cardiac output. In ECMO patients, increases in MAP may be achieved by increasing VA ECMO flows or by increasing SVR with vasopressors.

Maintain Pulsatility

VA ECMO has beneficial effects on the failing heart. Removing blood from the venous system leads to decreased preload, and, in turn, decreased LV end-diastolic volume and pressure and improved LV perfusion. These benefits are offset to varying degrees by the increase in afterload from the return of blood into the arterial system. Patients with poor cardiac contractility may be unable to eject against this afterload mismatch. When this occurs, the LV can become overdistended, leading to myocardial ischemia, as well as pulmonary edema or hemorrhage. In addition, blood may stagnate in the LV or aortic root, leading to thrombosis.[7] This issue can typically be detected by absence of pulsatility on the arterial waveform tracing. It can also be confirmed through echocardiography, which reveals LV distention and failure of the aortic valve to open.

There are several ways to offset the complications of afterload mismatch. Inotropic support can be used to augment contractility. In addition, VA ECMO flows can be reduced. Caution should be exercised when reducing ECMO flows to ensure that adequate tissue perfusion is maintained. Mechanical means of addressing this issue are sometimes used as well. Placement of an intra-aortic balloon pump can both augment coronary perfusion and reduce afterload. Alternatively, a percutaneous LVAD can be placed to facilitate LV decompression.[41] In addition, direct LV decompression can be achieved by placing a decompression cannula into the pulmonary artery, LA, or LV that drains directly to the inflow cannula of the ECMO circuit.[42]

Arrhythmias can compromise native cardiac function and should be addressed promptly. Antiarrhythmic medications, cardioversion, or pacing may be required.

Ensure Adequate Gas Exchange

The net systemic arterial oxygen content in ECMO patients is determined by contributions from both the native cardiac output and the output of the ECMO circuit. The relative contribution of the native cardiac output to systemic oxygenation varies based on both pulmonary status and myocardial function. As mentioned earlier, regional variation in arterial oxygen content can be seen, particularly in patients with femoral arterial cannulation. In patients with poor myocardial contractility, retrograde blood flow from the VA ECMO circuit to the aortic arch ensures adequate oxygen delivery to the coronary and cerebral circulation. However, as patients recover and regain myocardial function, the upper body may receive a substantial proportion of their blood flow from the native circulation. If patients have poor lung function this may result in delivery of poorly oxygenated blood to the upper body. Adequacy of systemic oxygenation should be assessed from an arterial cannula far removed from the influx of blood by the ECMO circuit to the arterial system. **Table 3** lists the recommended location of arterial blood gas sampling based on the location of the arterial cannula.

Extracorporeal Membrane Oxygenation Circuit

The ECMO circuit can regulate both oxygenation and ventilation. Oxygen delivery can be increased by increasing the fraction of delivered oxygen on the oxygen blender or increasing ECMO flow rates. Increased flow rates expose a greater blood volume to the membrane oxygenator, leading to greater oxygen delivery. Carbon dioxide removal is facilitated by the countercurrent sweep gas. Increasing the sweep gas flow rate results in more carbon dioxide removal. Alterations in ECMO blood flow rates do not affect carbon dioxide clearance.

Ventilator Management

To develop an appropriate mechanical ventilator strategy, clinicians must understand the physiologic consequences of positive pressure ventilation (PPV). PPV can be detrimental in the setting of RV failure caused by increased RV afterload.[43] In contrast, increased positive end-expiratory pressure (PEEP) may be beneficial in the setting of LV failure in which the increase in intrathoracic pressure leads to decreases in both LV preload and afterload.[44] Our practice is therefore to avoid high PEEP in patients with predominately RV failure. In patients with severely depressed LV function, we use moderate amounts of PEEP, because the increase in PEEP has beneficial hemodynamic effects and may help combat the development of pulmonary edema.[45–48] This issue is further addressed in respiratory strategies (See Bharat Awsare and colleagues' article, "Management strategies for Severe Respiratory Failure: as Extracorporeal Membrane Oxygenation (ECMO) is being considered," in this issue).

Monitoring Adequacy of Perfusion

Careful monitoring is required to ensure adequacy of ECMO support. Patients with adequate perfusion on stable ECMO settings can rapidly and subtly develop inadequacy of support for several reasons, including worsening pulmonary status, improving native cardiac function, anemia, arrhythmia, or deteriorating oxygenator membrane function. Most programs use ECMO specialists to monitor patients around the clock. Monitoring and frequent laboratory draws are used to detect changes and adjust support appropriately.

Flow meters on the circuit provide a continuous display of ECMO circuit outflows. Pressure monitors on the inflow cannula can detect excessive suction and ensure adequacy of venous drainage.[4] Inlet pressures should not be lower than −50 mm Hg.[7] Near-infrared spectroscopy can be used to detect changes in cerebral or limb perfusion.[49] These devices display a continuous read-out of tissue oxygen saturation (Sto_2).[50] Changes in the Sto_2 may detect alteration in perfusion, which can prompt early investigation and correction.

Mixed venous oxygen saturation (Svo_2) provides information regarding the balance between oxygen delivery and oxygen consumption. A normal Svo_2 is 65% to 75%. A low Svo_2 can be seen with either inadequate delivery of oxygen to tissues or a state of increased extraction.[51] Although a true Svo_2 cannot be measured in patients on VA ECMO, a sample from blood flow entering the circuit through the venous inflow cannula provides a reasonable surrogate.[7] When a low Svo_2 is observed on a prepump arterial blood gas measurement, it may reflect inadequacy of ECMO support. Possible corrective actions include increasing ECMO circuit flows to increase oxygen delivery or red blood cell transfusion to increase oxygen carrying capacity of the blood. Measurement of lactate level may be useful as well. There is increasing recognition that lactate level is not always simply a marker of inadequate perfusion and anaerobic metabolism but can also be caused by a hypermetabolic state caused by beta-2 stimulation and enhanced glycolysis.[52] Regardless of the cause, increase of plasma lactate levels seem to be associated with adverse ouctomes.[53] The authors think it is reasonable to periodically check lactate levels in VA ECMO patients. If increased levels are found, evaluation should be undertaken to assess for local (gut, limb) or global ischemia.

Hemoglobin Concentration

Historically, it was recommended that patients on ECMO support be transfused to near normal hemoglobin levels.[54] However, multiple studies in the general critical care population have shown no evidence of harm, and potential benefit from a restrictive transfusion strategy.[55] Limited data regarding transfusion practices exist in the ECMO population. Two small retrospective series specifically on ECMO patients showed no evidence of harm with restrictive transfusion strategies.[54,56] It is our practice to follow a restrictive transfusion strategy. Patients are typically maintained at a hematocrit greater than 25% and transfused only for bleeding or signs of inadequate oxygen delivery if above this threshold.

Anticoagulation and Bleeding

Significant disturbances of the coagulation system occur during extracorporeal support, leaving the patients vulnerable to both thrombosis and bleeding. Exposure of blood to the artificial surface of the ECMO circuit results in inflammation, cellular activation, and initiation of coagulation. In addition, turbulence and sheer stress compound this activation of coagulation and can lead to platelet and fibrin deposition.[57] Because of the alterations in hemostasis during ECMO support, anticoagulation is required to prevent thrombosis and preserve the patency of the circuit. Unfractionated heparin is most commonly used, although direct thrombin inhibitors are sometimes used as an alternative.[57] No consensus exists as to the optimal monitoring strategy or therapeutic range. Activating clotting time is the most widely used monitoring tool. Alternatives include the anti-Xa activity and activated partial thrombin time. Our center uses an anti-Xa–based strategy targeting a goal range of 0.3 to 0.5IU/mL. Fresh frozen plasma and cryoprecipitate transfusions are given to correct the International Normalized Ratio (INR) to less than 1.5 and fibrinogen level to greater than 100 mg/dL.[58] The authors typically transfuse platelets to maintain the count at more than 50 cells/mm^3; however, no consensus on the optimal transfusion threshold for platelets exists.

Bleeding complications are common, occurring in more than 20% of cases of VA ECMO support.[8] The severity of the bleeding dictates the response. Minor cannula site bleeding can be treated with hemostatic dressings or direct pressure. The cannula should also be examined to ensure it is properly positioned. The intensity of anticoagulation can be decreased and non–heparin-induced alterations in coagulation corrected (eg, fresh frozen plasma for increased INR). Antifibrinolytic therapy, such as aminocaproic or tranexamic acid, can be used as well. Severe bleeding may require surgical intervention and temporary cessation of anticoagulation. Recombinant factor VIIa use has been reported for uncontrollable bleeding in patients on ECMO.[59]

SUMMARY

VA ECMO can provide robust, highly customizable cardiac and pulmonary support for several conditions. It is likely that use of this powerful tool will continue to expand, so it is prudent for clinicians to familiarize themselves with its components and basic management strategies.

REFERENCES

1. Hill JD, O'Brien TG, Murray JJ, et al. Prolonged extracorporeal oxygenation for acute post-traumatic respiratory failure (shock-lung syndrome). Use of the Bramson membrane lung. N Engl J Med 1972;286(12):629–34.
2. Karagiannidis C, Brodie D, Strassmann S, et al. Extracorporeal membrane oxygenation: evolving epidemiology and mortality. Intensive Care Med 2016; 42(5):889–96.
3. Available at: http://www.elso.org/Registry/Statistics.aspx. Accessed February 4, 2017.
4. Lequier L, Horton SB, McMullan DM, et al. Extracorporeal membrane oxygenation circuitry. Pediatr Crit Care Med 2013;14(5 Suppl 1):S7–12.
5. MacLaren G, Combes A, Bartlett RH. Contemporary extracorporeal membrane oxygenation for adult respiratory failure: life support in the new era. Intensive Care Med 2012;38(2):210–20.

6. Napp LC, Kuhn C, Hoeper MM, et al. Cannulation strategies for percutaneous extracorporeal membrane oxygenation in adults. Clin Res Cardiol 2016;105(4): 283–96.

7. Chung M, Shiloh AL, Carlese A. Monitoring of the adult patient on venoarterial extracorporeal membrane oxygenation. ScientificWorldJournal 2014;2014: 393258.

8. Ventetuolo CE, Muratore CS. Extracorporeal life support in critically ill adults. Am J Respir Crit Care Med 2014;190(5):497–508.

9. Lim HS, Howell N, Ranasinghe A. Extracorporeal life support: physiological concepts and clinical outcomes. J Card Fail 2017;23(2):181–96.

10. Cheng R, Hachamovitch R, Kittleson M, et al. Clinical outcomes in fulminant myocarditis requiring extracorporeal membrane oxygenation: a weighted meta-analysis of 170 patients. J Card Fail 2014;20(6):400–6.

11. Ouweneel DM, Schotborgh JV, Limpens J, et al. Extracorporeal life support during cardiac arrest and cardiogenic shock: a systematic review and meta-analysis. Intensive Care Med 2016;42(12):1922–34.

12. Fukuhara S, Takeda K, Garan AR, et al. Contemporary mechanical circulatory support therapy for postcardiotomy shock. Gen Thorac Cardiovasc Surg 2016; 64(4):183–91.

13. Schmidt M, Burrell A, Roberts L, et al. Predicting survival after ECMO for refractory cardiogenic shock: the survival after veno-arterial-ECMO (SAVE)-score. Eur Heart J 2015;36(33):2246–56.

14. Conrad SA, Rycus PT. Extracorporeal membrane oxygenation for refractory cardiac arrest. Ann Card Anaesth 2017;20(Suppl):S4–10.

15. Wang GN, Chen XF, Qiao L, et al. Comparison of extracorporeal and conventional cardiopulmonary resuscitation: a meta-analysis of 2 260 patients with cardiac arrest. World J Emerg Med 2017;8(1):5–11.

16. Kagawa E. Extracorporeal cardiopulmonary resuscitation for adult cardiac arrest patients. World J Crit Care Med 2012;1(2):46–9.

17. Yusuff HO, Zochios V, Vuylsteke A. Extracorporeal membrane oxygenation in acute massive pulmonary embolism: a systematic review. Perfusion 2015;30(8): 611–6.

18. Dunne B, Christou E, Duff O, et al. Extracorporeal-assisted rewarming in the management of accidental deep hypothermic cardiac arrest: a systematic review of the literature. Heart Lung Circ 2014;23(11):1029–35.

19. Huang CT, Tsai YJ, Tsai PR, et al. Extracorporeal membrane oxygenation resuscitation in adult patients with refractory septic shock. J Thorac Cardiovasc Surg 2013;146(5):1041–6.

20. Park TK, Yang JH, Jeon K, et al. Extracorporeal membrane oxygenation for refractory septic shock in adults. Eur J Cardiothorac Surg 2015;47(2):e68–74.

21. Cheng A, Sun HY, Tsai MS, et al. Predictors of survival in adults undergoing extracorporeal membrane oxygenation with severe infections. J Thorac Cardiovasc Surg 2016;152(6):1526–36.e1.

22. Brechot N, Luyt CE, Schmidt M, et al. Venoarterial extracorporeal membrane oxygenation support for refractory cardiovascular dysfunction during severe bacterial septic shock. Crit Care Med 2013;41(7):1616–26.

23. Abrams D, Brodie D. Novel uses of extracorporeal membrane oxygenation in adults. Clin Chest Med 2015;36(3):373–84.

24. de Lange DW, Sikma MA, Meulenbelt J. Extracorporeal membrane oxygenation in the treatment of poisoned patients. Clin Toxicol (Phila) 2013;51(5):385–93.

25. Tseng YH, Wu TI, Liu YC, et al. Venoarterial extracorporeal life support in post-traumatic shock and cardiac arrest: lessons learned. Scand J Trauma Resusc Emerg Med 2014;22:12.

26. Weiss GM, Fandrick AD, Sidebotham D. Successful rescue of an adult with refractory anaphylactic shock and abdominal compartment syndrome with venoarterial extracorporeal membrane oxygenation and bedside laparotomy. Semin Cardiothorac Vasc Anesth 2015;19(1):66–70.

27. Dolmatova E, Moazzami K, Cocke TP, et al. Extracorporeal membrane oxygenation in transcatheter aortic valve replacement. Asian Cardiovasc Thorac Ann 2017;25(1):31–4.

28. Broman LM, Holzgraefe B, Palmer K, et al. The Stockholm experience: interhospital transports on extracorporeal membrane oxygenation. Crit Care 2015;19:278.

29. Reeb J, Olland A, Renaud S, et al. Vascular access for extracorporeal life support: tips and tricks. J Thorac Dis 2016;8(Suppl 4):S353–63.

30. Ghodsizad A, Koerner MM, Brehm CE, et al. The role of extracorporeal membrane oxygenation circulatory support in the 'crash and burn' patient: from implantation to weaning. Curr Opin Cardiol 2014;29(3):275–80.

31. Rupprecht L, Lunz D, Philipp A, et al. Pitfalls in percutaneous ECMO cannulation. Heart Lung Vessel 2015;7(4):320–6.

32. Jayaraman AL, Cormican D, Shah P, et al. Cannulation strategies in adult venoarterial and veno-venous extracorporeal membrane oxygenation: techniques, limitations, and special considerations. Ann Card Anaesth 2017;20(Suppl):S11–8.

33. Lamb KM, Hirose H, Cavarocchi NC. Preparation and technical considerations for percutaneous cannulation for veno-arterial extracorporeal membrane oxygenation. J Card Surg 2013;28(2):190–2.

34. Biscotti M, Bacchetta M. The "sport model": extracorporeal membrane oxygenation using the subclavian artery. Ann Thorac Surg 2014;98(4):1487–9.

35. Takayama H, Landes E, Truby L, et al. Feasibility of smaller arterial cannulas in venoarterial extracorporeal membrane oxygenation. J Thorac Cardiovasc Surg 2015;149(5):1428–33.

36. Cove ME, MacLaren G. Clinical review: mechanical circulatory support for cardiogenic shock complicating acute myocardial infarction. Crit Care 2010;14(5):235.

37. Herlihy JP, Loyalka P, Jayaraman G, et al. Extracorporeal membrane oxygenation using the TandemHeart System's catheters. Tex Heart Inst J 2009;36(4):337–41.

38. Gilotra NA, Stevens GR. Temporary mechanical circulatory support: a review of the options, indications, and outcomes. Clin Med Insights Cardiol 2014;8(Suppl 1):75–85.

39. Vincent JL, De Backer D. Inotrope/vasopressor support in sepsis-induced organ hypoperfusion. Semin Respir Crit Care Med 2001;22(1):61–74.

40. D'Aragon F, Belley-Cote EP, Meade MO, et al. Blood pressure targets for vasopressor therapy: a systematic review. Shock 2015;43(6):530–9.

41. Koeckert MS, Jorde UP, Naka Y, et al. Impella LP 2.5 for left ventricular unloading during venoarterial extracorporeal membrane oxygenation support. J Card Surg 2011;26(6):666–8.

42. Weymann A, Schmack B, Sabashnikov A, et al. Central extracorporeal life support with left ventricular decompression for the treatment of refractory cardiogenic shock and lung failure. J Cardiothorac Surg 2014;9:60.

43. King C, May CW, Williams J, et al. Management of right heart failure in the critically ill. Crit Care Clin 2014;30(3):475–98.

44. Buda AJ, Pinsky MR, Ingels NB Jr, et al. Effect of intrathoracic pressure on left ventricular performance. N Engl J Med 1979;301(9):453–9.

45. Schmidt M, Pellegrino V, Combes A, et al. Mechanical ventilation during extracorporeal membrane oxygenation. Crit Care 2014;18(1):203.

46. Acute Respiratory Distress Syndrome Network, Brower RG, Matthay MA, Morris A, et al. Ventilation with lower tidal volumes as compared with traditional tidal volumes for acute lung injury and the acute respiratory distress syndrome. The Acute Respiratory Distress Syndrome Network. N Engl J Med 2000; 342(18):1301–8.

47. Putensen C, Theuerkauf N, Zinserling J, et al. Meta-analysis: ventilation strategies and outcomes of the acute respiratory distress syndrome and acute lung injury. Ann Intern Med 2009;151(8):566–76.

48. Gattinoni L, Tonetti T, Quintel M. How best to set the ventilator on extracorporeal membrane lung oxygenation. Curr Opin Crit Care 2017;23(1):66–72.

49. Wong JK, Smith TN, Pitcher HT, et al. Cerebral and lower limb near-infrared spectroscopy in adults on extracorporeal membrane oxygenation. Artif Organs 2012; 36(8):659–67.

50. Scheeren TW, Schober P, Schwarte LA. Monitoring tissue oxygenation by near infrared spectroscopy (NIRS): background and current applications. J Clin Monit Comput 2012;26(4):279–87.

51. Walley KR. Use of central venous oxygen saturation to guide therapy. Am J Respir Crit Care Med 2011;184(5):514–20.

52. Levy B. Lactate and shock state: the metabolic view. Curr Opin Crit Care 2006; 12(4):315–21.

53. Jung C, Janssen K, Kaluza M, et al. Outcome predictors in cardiopulmonary resuscitation facilitated by extracorporeal membrane oxygenation. Clin Res Cardiol 2016;105(3):196–205.

54. Voelker MT, Busch T, Bercker S, et al. Restrictive transfusion practice during extracorporeal membrane oxygenation therapy for severe acute respiratory distress syndrome. Artif Organs 2015;39(4):374–8.

55. Carson JL, Carless PA, Hebert PC. Transfusion thresholds and other strategies for guiding allogeneic red blood cell transfusion. Cochrane Database Syst Rev 2012;(4):CD002042.

56. Agerstrand CL, Burkart KM, Abrams DC, et al. Blood conservation in extracorporeal membrane oxygenation for acute respiratory distress syndrome. Ann Thorac Surg 2015;99(2):590–5.

57. Andrews J, Winkler AM. Challenges with navigating the precarious hemostatic balance during extracorporeal life support: implications for coagulation and transfusion management. Transfus Med Rev 2016;30(4):223–9.

58. Available at: https://www.elso.org/Portals/0/Files/elsoanticoagulationguideline8-2014-table-contents.pdf. Accessed February 16, 2017.

59. Repesse X, Au SM, Brechot N, et al. Recombinant factor VIIa for uncontrollable bleeding in patients with extracorporeal membrane oxygenation: report on 15 cases and literature review. Crit Care 2013;17(2):R55.

Management Strategies for Severe Respiratory Failure

As Extracorporeal Membrane Oxygenation Is Being Considered

Bharat Awsare, MD, Justin Herman, MD, Michael Baram, MD*

KEYWORDS

- Respiratory failure • ARDS • ECMO • Multiorgan failure • Mechanical ventilation

KEY POINTS

- ARDS is an inflammatory disease that is perpetuated by ventilator-induced lung injury (VILI).
- ECMO offers an opportunity for ultraprotective lung protection and rest.
- Utility of ECMO is determined by disease cause and reversibility.
- Initiation of ECMO requires an organized, preplanned, coordinated effort.

INTRODUCTION

The role of extracorporeal membrane oxygenation (ECMO) in the management of severe respiratory failure continues to evolve as increases in gained institutional experience and improvements in technology transform opinions regarding its utility.[1–6] Since the H1N1 influenza pandemic of 2009, the use of ECMO for severe respiratory failure has been on the rise.[2,7,8] This article facilitates the efficient coordination of care of the potential ECMO patient among the multidisciplinary members of the ECMO team. The exact parameters determining the ideal ECMO candidate have yet to be identified.[9] Numerous scoring systems exist to identify potential benefiters from this invasive technology.[10–12] There is no exact definition of severe respiratory failure; however, the Murray score, which is defined by oxygenation, positive end-expiratory pressure needs, compliance, and chest radiography, remains the gold standard.[13] There is

No author has any commercial or financial conflicts of interest or funding sources related to this article.

Division of Pulmonary and Critical Care Medicine, Department of Medicine, Thomas Jefferson University, 834 Walnut Street, Suite 650, Philadelphia, PA 19107, USA

* Corresponding author.

E-mail address: Michael.Baram@jefferson.edu

no standard of care for the potential pre-ECMO patient with severe respiratory failure. Individual institutions should develop a multidisciplinary algorithm of management based on local resources, expertise, and opinions.[1,14,15] It is crucial for the team to set realistic expectations regarding ECMO candidacy and provide guidelines as to what levels of physiologic failure ECMO should be considered, initiated, or deemed futile.

Although early evidence from the late 1970s demonstrated no benefit in ECMO support, improvements in the understanding of acute respiratory distress syndrome (ARDS), ventilator management, and ECMO technology has been a game-changer.[16–18] Webb and Tierney[19] described lung inflammation and injury induced by the ventilator termed ventilator-induced lung injury (VILI). Understanding that ARDS is an inflammatory process is the key to overcoming it, and the subsequent multiorgan failure (MOF) that it causes.[20] Critical to the management of ARDS is to minimize continued lung injury.[21,22] The classic ARDS Network paper set the current gold standard of minimizing VILI by reducing volutrauma.[23,24] Additionally, multiple randomized studies support lower mortality with lower tidal volume ventilation.[25] The biologic plausibility for this may be lower cytokine levels, which decrease incidence of multiple organ system failure.[26] ARDS survivors show reductions in measured proinflammatory cytokines.[27,28] When ECMO is used, it is clear that ECMO itself is not the cause of improved cytokine levels; in fact, the initiation ECMO can initially increase inflammation.[29] ECMO does provide the opportunity for implementing a low stretch lung strategy and low driving pressure, which reduces VILI.[15,17,30–32] The reduction of high fractional inspired oxygen (F_{IO_2}) provides another mechanism of ECMO benefit.[33,34] The basic premise of ECMO support is that it provides an opportunity for lung rest in the setting of ARDS.[17,31,35] Overall, ECMO serves as a means to reduce VILI, which can worsen ARDS.[20,36,37] The idea of "lung stress" is an emerging concept in mechanical ventilation in ARDS. Increases in lung stress as measured by driving pressure (plateau pressure minus positive end-expiratory pressure) have been associated with worse outcomes in ARDS.[38] Driving pressures of 15 cm H_2O or higher were associated with poor outcomes and may identify a subset of patients for whom ECMO may be indicated. Serpa Neto and colleagues[39] studied outcomes of ECMO based on ventilator settings and found driving pressure to be the only ventilator setting associated with hospital mortality.

When to initiate ECMO as a means to prevent VILI and provide lung rest is unclear.[40,41] Early ventilator trauma can be identified in pre-ARDS, and strategies to reduce early cytokine release to avoid unbridled inflammation have led to a belief that initiation of ECMO after 7 days is not indicated.[31,42,43] Proponents of early ECMO believe the complication and severity of MOF is mitigated by early cannulation; however, no randomized, prospective human studies exist to compare timing of cannulation.[44–46] An observational study demonstrated that early cannulation led to a risk reduction of death, but a longer length of hospital stay. A small sheep study in ARDS induced by smoke failed to show advantage of early ECMO.[47] It is known that organ failure can recover on ECMO, but whether early ECMO prevents MOF is unclear.[48] However, it is clear that prolonged mechanical ventilation pre-ECMO does have worse outcomes.[35,49,50] Pranikoff and colleagues conducted a retrospective study that exhibited that mortality correlated with duration of time in respiratory failure precannnulation. The CESAR trial revealed that a coordinated effort of identification of ARDS patients and transfer to centers that are ECMO-capable improves outcomes.[43] This benefit likely extended beyond simply initiating patients on ECMO, because centers with high volume of ARDS and ECMO capabilities have improved outcomes.[6,51]

INDICATIONS FOR EXTRACORPOREAL MEMBRANE OXYGENATION

ECMO is indicated for the support of pulmonary function in acute respiratory failure until native pulmonary function is restored, or in chronic respiratory failure as a bridge to transplantation. The Extracorporeal Life Support Organization, which registers ECMO usage, has documented nearly 20,000 usages of ECMO in adults from 1985 to 2015 with approximately 9000 usages for respiratory indications.[52] This section focuses on the common indications for venous-venous (VV)-ECMO.

Acute Respiratory Distress Syndrome

ARDS is the most common respiratory indication for ECMO, and the respiratory indication for which there is the highest level of evidence. ARDS may be caused by diverse conditions, such as pneumonia, sepsis, inhalational injury, pancreatitis, trauma, lung contusion, and through distinct mechanisms that cause epithelial and/or endothelial injury. ECMO is used in ARDS to correct hypoxemia and respiratory acidosis and to provide lung protection from VILI. Registries in Italy and Australia showed a survival of 68% and 71%, respectively, in patients with ARDS caused by H1N1 influenza treated with ECMO.[53,54]

According to Extracorporeal Life Support Organization guidelines, ECMO should be considered in severe hypoxic respiratory failure when the expected mortality rate is greater than 50% as evidenced by a Pao_2/Fio_2 ratio less than 150 on an Fio_2 greater than 90% and a Murray Score of 2 to 3. ECMO is indicated when the expected mortality rate is greater than 80% as evidenced by a Pao_2/Fio_2 ratio less than 100 on an Fio_2 greater than 90% and a Murray Score of 3 to 4 despite optimal care for 6 hours or more.[37] The CESAR trial, which reintroduced the applicability of ECMO as a support tool for ARDS, used the Murray score to help define respiratory failure. The indications for ECMO in the CESAR trial included severe potentially reversible respiratory failure in patients on mechanical ventilation less than 7 days, Murray score greater than 2.5, or uncompensated hypercapnia with pH less than 7.20.[43] The PRESERVE score and the RESP score are two tools to help predict survivability on ECMO.[10,12] Although these tools have flaws, they may help identify patients who have poor outcomes with ECMO. This topic is discussed further later.

Contraindications for the use of ECMO in ARDS are generally center-specific, but generally consist of anatomic considerations (morbid obesity, difficult anatomy for cannulation) and clinical considerations (mechanical ventilation >7 days, coagulopathy or contraindications to anticoagulation, immunosuppression, malignancy on active chemotherapy, stem cell transplantation, pulmonary fibrosis, and poor prognosis caused by comorbidities or neurologic insult).[5] Ultimately, deciding when the stress of conventional mechanical ventilation to achieve gas exchange and limit airway injury is higher than the risks of extracorporeal life support drives the decision to initiate ECMO on an individual patient basis.

At our institution, criteria for ECMO are not only based on conventional indications and contraindications, but also are modified based on prior institutional experience with multispecialty input. ECMO is generally considered in younger patients, cases of potentially reversible respiratory failure, and onset of mechanical ventilation less than 7 days. Relative contraindications are body mass index greater than 45, poor neurologic prognosis, contraindications to anticoagulation, immunosuppression, bacteremia, vasculitis, pulmonary fibrosis, MOF, and presence of a patent foramen ovale (PFO; caused by the risk of paradoxic systemic emboli). Ultimately final decisions regarding ECMO initiation are made in a multispecialty fashion on a case-to-case basis after discussion of all the previously mentioned considerations.

Lung Transplantation

The use of ECMO as a bridge to transplantation increased dramatically after 2009.[55] Four cohort studies published demonstrated successful bridging to transplantation of 74% to 89% in 123 patients with ECMO mean durations of 4 to 14 days.[56–59] ECMO also has been used as supportive therapy for patients after lung transplantation including patients with primary graft failure.[60] Indications for initiating ECMO vary by center, but generally involve younger patients with single organ failure who have the greatest chance of rehabilitation after transplant.[61] Another application in this subset is the use of ECMO in nonintubated patients with end-stage lung disease as a bridge to transplant.[62]

Miscellaneous

ECMO and extracorporeal CO_2 removal have been used in a variety of other pulmonary disorders to support gas exchange or limit the effects of mechanical ventilation on a case-series basis for respiratory failure in obstructive lung disease, diffuse alveolar hemorrhage, and severe air leak syndromes. However, the evidence for these uses is still preliminary at best and therefore they have not been widely adopted.

The most promising of these indications may be the use of extracorporeal CO_2 removal in acute exacerbations of chronic obstructive pulmonary disease with hypercapnic respiratory failure as a means of avoiding invasive mechanical ventilation. A pilot study showed that CO_2 removal was feasible through a single catheter using low flows.[63] In addition to the clinical implications of avoiding mechanical ventilation, there is a potential of cost savings through the decrease of intensive care unit (ICU) and hospital length of stay.[64]

There are also case reports of ECMO being used for inhalation and occupational injury, severe bleeding from lung injury tracheal injury, and to support patients through complex respiratory procedures.[65,66]

APPROACH TO THE VENTILATOR PRE–EXTRACORPOREAL MEMBRANE OXYGENATION
Lung-Protective Strategy

No single ventilation strategy has been proven as the best bridge to ECMO. The lung-protective ventilation strategy was solidified as the standard for prevention of VILI after the ARDSnet group's publication of the ARMA study in 2000.[26] This study compared a traditional tidal volume of 12 mL/kg of predicted body weight and a plateau pressure less than or equal to 50 cm H_2O, to a low tidal volume of 6 mL/kg predicted body weight and a plateau pressure of less than or equal to 30 cm H_2O in 861 mechanically ventilated patients with ARDS. Despite having initially worse oxygenation, the low tidal volume group was found to have an 8.8% absolute reduction in mortality (39.8% vs 31.0%; $P = .007$), more ventilator-free days (10 vs 12; $P = .007$), and more days free of extrapulmonary organ failure (12 vs 15; $P = .006$).[26] Additional studies have also demonstrated that this strategy improves outcomes if adopted earlier in the course of ARDS, and that there is a mortality benefit at 2 years.[67,68] With a volume-limited ventilatory strategy, some degree of respiratory acidosis develops despite attempts to maintain minute ventilation with increased respiratory rates. For example, Hickling and colleagues[69] reported a mean $Paco_2$ of 67 torr and a mean pH of 7.2 when using a lung-protective ventilation strategy in ARDS patients. Providers must permit some degree of hypercapnia, in order for their patient's to reap the survival benefits that were demonstrated in the ARMA study. If a satisfactory balance between oxygenation, ventilation, and hemodynamics cannot be achieved (even with medical comanagement, discussed later) clinicians may change modes. Unfortunately, despite their theoretic benefits, the clinical evidence supporting alternative ventilator techniques is lacking. The decision to revert to ECMO therapy remains on the balance of strategies that improve oxygenation versus ventilation. Once an oxygenation strategy severely worsens ventilation, and vice versa, ECMO should be considered.

Airway Pressure Release Ventilation and High-Frequency Oscillatory Ventilation

Modes other than assist control ventilation have been used in ARDS. Airway pressure release ventilation (APRV) provides continuous positive airway pressure while cycling between high and a low pressure level at set time intervals, and allows for spontaneous breaths at both pressure levels. Most of the observed benefits seen in APRV are attributable to the ability of patients to take spontaneous breaths. As a result this mode should not be used in patients requiring deep sedation or neuromuscular blockade (NMB), which is common in severe ARDS.[70] There have been few randomized controlled trials to evaluate APRV in ARDS, and the studies that were published had small sample sizes, failed to compare APRV with standard practices in mechanical ventilation for ARDS, and they yielded conflicting results.[70–75] Therefore there is inadequate evidence to recommend for or against the use of APRV in patients with ARDS. A common clinical confounder with APRV are the recommendations of early paralytics, which precludes the use of APRV.

High-frequency oscillatory ventilation (HFOV) is a mode of ventilation that uses high-frequency fluctuations in pressure via an oscillator to deliver low tidal volume breaths at a rapid rate while maintaining a constant mean airway pressure. This mode initially seemed like it would be the ideal strategy to prevent VILI in ARDS; however, two prospective, randomized, multicenter trials that were published in 2013 demonstrated no benefit. The OSCILLATE trial published by Ferguson and colleagues[76] compared HFOV with a standard lung-protective ventilation strategy in 548 patients with moderate-severe ARDS. In-hospital mortality was higher in the HFOV group when compared with the control group (47% vs 35%; relative risk [RR] of death with HFOV, 1.33; 95% confidence interval [CI], 1.09–1.64; $P = .005$), and the HFOV group received more vasopressors, NMB, and sedatives than the control group.[76] The OSCAR trial by Young and colleagues[77] came to similar conclusions when comparing HFOV with usual care in 398 patients with moderate-severe ARDS. The overall 30-day mortality was similar in the HFOV group compared with the control group (41.7% vs 41.1%), and the HFOV group again received more vasopressors and paralytics than the control group.[77] Based on these two trials, HFOV cannot be routinely recommended for use in ARDS. At our institution, usage of adult HFOV has significantly declined after the OSCILLATE and OSCAR trials revealed no benefit and possible harm.

Medical Supportive Therapies

Corticosteroids

Because ARDS is an inflammatory lung injury, one would expect that corticosteroids would be an ideal treatment modality. The 2006 ARDS network study published by Steinberg and colleagues[78] was a multicenter randomized controlled trial that compared methylprednisolone with placebo in 180 patients who had ARDS for at least 7 days with a primary end point of 60-day mortality. The 60-day hospital mortality rate was 28.6% in the placebo group (95% CI, 20.3%–38.6%) and 29.2% in the methylprednisolone group (95% CI, 20.8%–39.4%; $P = 1.0$). Additionally, methylprednisolone was associated with significantly increased 60-day and 180-day mortality rates for patients enrolled at least 14 days after the onset of ARDS. Based on these findings, the authors concluded that corticosteroids could not be recommended for use in persistent ARDS, and that corticosteroids may actually cause harm in certain subgroups of patients.[78]

Ruan and colleagues[79] published a meta-analysis of eight randomized controlled trials and 10 cohort studies in 2014 that examined the effects of corticosteroids in ARDS. The randomized controlled trials demonstrated that steroids had a statistically insignificant effect on ICU mortality (RR, 0.55; 95% CI, 0.24–1.25) and no effect on 60-day mortality (RR, 0.97; 95% CI, 0.75–1.26). A subgroup analysis by cause of the ARDS demonstrated that steroids significantly increased mortality in influenza-related ARDS (RR, 2.45; 95% CI, 1.40–4.27).[79] Given that ARDS is a syndrome that is caused by multiple etiologies, it is not surprising that there is a heterogeneous response to steroids in patients with ARDS reported in the literature. For instance, in pneumocystis pneumonia or diffuse alveolar hemorrhage related–ARDS, steroids would be expected to have a positive response, because steroids are part of the usual therapy in these underlying conditions. However, in undifferentiated ARDS and influenza-related ARDS, the current literature does not support use of corticosteroids.[78,79] Although Pao_2/Fio_2 ratios do improve with steroids, this is not reflected in improved outcomes. The same evidence can be applied to steroid use for patients with ARDS being considered for ECMO. If steroids are being used as a short-term buffer to avoid ECMO, it seems that it takes 48 hours to see a significant effect from methylprednisolone on ARDS.[80]

Diuretics

In the setting of lung injury, small increases in the pulmonary-artery occlusion pressure are associated with large increases in extravascular fluid in the lung.[81] In 2006, the ARDS Network group published a study comparing 60-day mortality when a liberal versus a conservative fluid management strategy was followed over a 7-day period in 1000 patients with acute lung injury.[82] It found significant differences in that the conservative strategy group had improved lung function, shorter durations of mechanical ventilation, and shorter ICU stays, without increases in extrapulmonary organ failure.[82] This study supports the use of diuretics to maintain a negative fluid balance in patients with ARDS. Of note, patients in the conservative group had lower hemodynamic measurements; however, this did not translate into increased vasopressor use or end-organ damage. Although diuretics have not been shown to improve mortality, they can improve lung function, reduce duration of mechanical ventilation, and decrease ICU length of stay in ARDS. With the rapid effects of diuretics, a trial of diuretics can be attempted to help avoid ECMO or to improve oxygenation as ECMO is being initiated.

Prone-positioning

Prone-positioning has been proposed as a method to improve chest-wall compliance, improve ventilation-perfusion matching, recruit dependent lung zones, decrease ventilator-associated pneumonia, and to more homogenously distribute lung strain in the setting of ARDS.[83] Early studies of prone-positioning in ARDS failed to demonstrate an overall survival benefit; however, subset analysis did demonstrate benefit in patients with the most severe hypoxia.[84,85] In 2013, Guerin and colleagues[86] published the PROSEVA trial, which evaluated the effects of prone-positioning in patients with moderate-severe ARDS. They found that the patients that were in the prone-position group had lower 28-day mortality compared with the supine-position group (16.0% vs 32.8%; P<.001). Additionally, they found that this difference in cumulative probability of survival developed within the first week of follow-up and persisted through 90 days.[86] A 2014 meta-analysis by Beitler and colleagues[87] examined the effects of prone-positioning in only the studies that used a lung-protective ventilation strategy (excluded studies where >8 mL/kg tidal volumes were used). This meta-analysis found that prone-positioning significantly reduced 60-day mortality from ARDS when used in conjunction with low-tidal-volume ventilation (RR of death, 0.66; 95% CI, 0.50–0.86; P = .002).[87] Based on these more recent studies, prone-positioning ought to be attempted in the setting of refractory hypoxia secondary to ARDS. Multiple studies have shown that the benefits of prone positioning can be seen within 24 hours.[88] This benefit must be balanced by the worse outcomes in delayed ECMO initiation.[49]

Vasodilators

Selective pulmonary vasodilators, such as inhaled nitric oxide (iNO) and inhaled epoprostenol (iEPO), are commonly used in cases of severe ARDS with refractory hypoxemia. Inhaled vasodilators deliver drug to areas of lung parenchyma capable of ventilation, thereby improving ventilation-perfusion mismatch, and improving hypoxemia.[89] A 2016 Cochrane review examined the effects of iNO on mortality in ARDS. It included 14 randomized controlled trials, with 1275 patients.[90] The authors concluded that although iNO improved oxygenation, it did not reduce morality in patients with ARDS, regardless of the severity of the hypoxemia, and that iNO actually increased the risk of renal failure in these patients.[90] In a retrospective, single-center study, iEPO was compared with iNO, and was found to not only be much less expensive but also noninferior to iNO in terms of improving oxygenation.[91] Prostacyclins, such as iEPO, also have additional effects secondary to their mechanism of action. Prostacyclins enhance the cyclic adenosine monophosphate axis, which leads to increased surfactant production and down-regulation of proinflammatory cytokines, both of which may provide additional benefit in the setting of ARDS.[92,93] Despite these promising physiologic effects and studies demonstrating improvements in hypoxia and hemodynamics (reduced pulmonary artery pressure without reducing mean arterial pressure or systemic vascular resistance) in the setting of ARDS, there is an almost complete lack of evidence demonstrating mortality benefit from use of iEPO in ARDS.[94] The 2010 Cochrane review of iEPO use in ARDS highlighted this lack of data demonstrating a mortality benefit.[95] They only found one randomized controlled trial, in a pediatric population, with a small sample size (n = 14) that examined mortality as a primary end point. The short half-life of this agent reduces the deleterious effects of iEPO. Its safety profile makes iEPO a standard therapy for transport and salvage to ECMO facilities.[96]

Neuromuscular blockade

In patients requiring mechanical ventilation, NMB can improve respiratory mechanics via elimination of the work of breathing, reduction of resistance from the chest wall and abdomen, and improvement in patient-ventilator synchrony. In 2004, Gainnier and colleagues[97] demonstrated that 48 hours of NMB with cisatracurium led to improved oxygenation in ARDS patients. The first trial to report a mortality benefit from NMB was the ACURASYS trial, which was published by Papazian and colleagues in 2010.[98] It was a multicenter randomized controlled trial involving 340 patients with severe ARDS that examined whether early initiation of NMB with cisatracurium resulted in an adjusted mortality benefit when compared with placebo (adjusted for baseline Pao_2/Fio_2 ratio, simplified acute physiology score, and plateau pressure). They reported a hazard ratio of death at 90 days of 0.68 (95% CI, 0.48–0.98; P = .04) for the NMB group. The crude 90-day mortality was 31.6% (95% CI, 25.2–38.8) in the cisatracurium group versus 40.7% (95% CI, 33.5–48.4) in the placebo group (P = .08).[98]

Unfortunately, the study was underpowered to show a statistically significant difference. However, the NMB group was found to have a significantly lower 28-day mortality rate, more ventilator-free days, more organ failure–free days, and lower rates of pneumothorax than the control group.[98] A 2013 meta-analysis of prior studies by Alhazzani and colleagues[99] reported a significant reduction in the crude all-cause mortality rate and lower rates of barotrauma without an increase in the rate of ICU-acquired weakness when cisatracurium was used early in the course of treatment of severe ARDS. However, it should be noted that all included studies were from the same group of investigators and not blinded. Given the available data, paralytics have been a mainstay of early management of severe acute respiratory failure. This is a therapy that is quickly initiated for a decompensating patient with effects that are rapidly seen.

PLANNING FOR EXTRACORPOREAL MEMBRANE OXYGENATION

Whether ARDS is being managed at a non-ECMO providing site or a referral site, consideration for ECMO support for ARDS should be done in a methodical, organized manner.[14] Interhospital teams have shown that transport of patients with severe respiratory failure can be safely done.[100] Centers with high ECMO volumes have improved outcomes.[101,102] Much of this benefit is because of the improved processes set into place; however, the reasons are multifactorial.[103] Because ARDS is often just one of the clinical manifestations of multiorgan dysfunction syndrome, other factors may affect the decisions for and logistics of ECMO, and they must be evaluated before cannulation. Cardiac function, comorbidities that increase the risk of hemorrhage, risk of active infection, history of vena cava filters, and clarification of goals of care and the assignment of a medical decision maker must all be clarified early in this process before moving forward with ECMO cannulation. All of this information must be clearly documented and communicated to the ECMO team to avoid errors and miscommunications.

Assessment of Cardiac Function

Although this article encompasses severe respiratory failure, assessing cardiac function is essential for determining ECMO options. If time permits, a pre-ECMO echocardiogram may affect plans.[104] VV-ECMO is designed to support failing lungs by providing a medium for gas exchange, but does little for circulatory support. Patients with ARDS often have right ventricular failure, but an echocardiogram can help determine if the right ventricular dysfunction is caused by hypoxemia and reactive pulmonary hypertension, or if it is a manifestation of global dysfunction.[105,106] McConnell sign, which is apical hyperactivity with hypokinesis of the remaining right ventricular, suggests acute strain but has multiple causes.[107] Cardiac output may improve with the initiation of VV-ECMO alone by improving oxygenation and ameliorating reactive pulmonary hypertension.[106] Global dysfunction may suggest that venous-arterial (VA)-ECMO may be needed to help in oxygenation, ventilation, and mechanical support of circulation.

There are other benefits to pre-ECMO echocardiogram. Aortic dissection, aortic regurgitation, and mitral regurgitation are relative contraindications to VA-ECMO.[104] The increased afterload from the ECMO pump would worsen left-sided valve dysfunction and could trigger congestive heart failure on top of ARDS. A color Doppler flow may identify a PFO, which raises multiple issues for VV-ECMO.[104] The pressure jet from the cannula may increase right-to-left shunting and allow air-emboli to travel to the left heart. In addition, a PFO may affect weaning and shunt fractions. Although a

PFO is not an absolute contraindication, it must be considered in the risk-benefit analysis because of this risk of stroke. A PFO may change the cannulation approach. The team may change to a dual-cannula approach rather than a single-cannula with a double lumen, which produces a flow jet aimed toward the cardiac septum and is deadly in the setting of a PFO.

Assessment for Sepsis

Understanding the bacterial load and lack of benefit of ECMO (VA and VV) in supporting vasodilatory shock may affect decision making. The interplay of ARDS and MOF with septic shock increases the complexity of hemodynamic monitoring and support. The large size of the cannulas used for VA and VV and the prolonged duration of ECMO runs (on average lasting around 9 days) put patients at risk for bacterial colonization and infection.[15,108] In the past, sepsis was a contraindication to ECMO; however, this is no longer the case.[109] There is literature that suggests surveillance cultures precannulation and postcannulation can identify occult bacteremia in 28% of patients.[110,111] Some sites report new infections could be 40%.[108] Depending on the scenario, these bacteremias are gram-positive skin organisms, candida species, or multidrug-resistant organisms. The probability of infection increased with length of ECMO, but did not seem to impact mortality.[112]

Our institution uses ECMO for patients with sepsis, but not for patients with active bacteremia. With evidence that pneumonia can often be associated with bacteremia, this makes decision making challenging. Our institution has adopted a liberal initiation policy. However, once cavitation is seen on imaging, our site often does not initiate ECMO because of the risks of high bacterial loads.

Assessment for an Inferior Vena Cava Filter

Our institution routinely images to assess for inferior vena cava filter filters for patients who may need femoral venous ECMO cannulation. If a filter is present, it can affect the placement of guidewires and cannulas via the femoral approach. Institutional experience has been improved with interventional radiology snaring removable filters and providing a safe vessel for cannulation.

Assessment for Central Nervous System Disease

Although not predictable in adult patients with respiratory failure, intracranial hemorrhage occurs roughly in 5%.[108] In mixed cases of ECMO (cardiac and pulmonary caused by hypoxia, or cardiovascular failure pre-ECMO or on pump), brain death has been reported in 7% to 21% of ECMO cases.[113] These data contain cardiovascular collapse and arrest so the causal incidence of central nervous system injury on VV-ECMO is not as well differentiated.

Clarification of Goals of Care

Family involvement in ECMO patients is important. Families must understand the commitment to prolonged support and long rehabilitation necessary to return patients to their previous quality of life. Our institutional experience has shown that more than 90% of the patients who survive VV-ECMO and the decannulation process survive to hospital discharge.[114] The correlate of this is also important. There sometimes reaches a point where MOF is persistent and the possibility of transition from ECMO is not possible or prognosis is poor because of neurologic complications. Families must be prepared to make end-of-life decisions and withdraw care despite preserved oxygenation and hemodynamics provided by the multiple forms of life support. Families must be educated about the level of support that VA-ECMO provides and that cardiopulmonary resuscitation on VA-ECMO would be futile. The ECMO team must have a good working relationship with families to ensure that they have realistic expectations about the limitations of this rescue therapy.

The PRESERV and RESP scoring tools can help predict who has a 90% likelihood of death on ECMO, and this information can help the medical team and patients' families make better informed decisions about when and when not to pursue ECMO cannulation for respiratory failure.[12] Given the heterogeneity of causes of respiratory failure, mixed age distribution of patients affected by ARDS, and emergency need for this therapy, the ECMO field remains at a loss for a perfect patient-selection tool.

SUMMARY

This article reviews much of the evidence for medical support in severe ARDS with signs of severe respiratory failure and/or MOF. ECMO provides a tool to allow lung rest and support an "ultra-low-volume" lung strategy.[15,17,30–32] Understanding the limits of what medical management can offer in this setting helps clinicians feel confident to use or withhold ECMO support in their patients with refractory hypoxemia. Traditionally VV-ECMO is considered as a tool for respiratory failure and VA-ECMO is a tool for cardiac support. There are scenarios where severe hypoxia causes acute cor pulmonale, which may cause a need for VA-ECMO in the setting of respiratory failure. The other articles in this issue follow the traditional lines: VV-ECMO is for acute lung failure and VA-ECMO is for cardiac support.

REFERENCES

1. Bellani G, Laffey JG, Pham T, et al. Epidemiology, patterns of care, and mortality for patients with acute respiratory distress syndrome in intensive care units in 50 countries. JAMA 2016;315(8):788–800.
2. Turner DA, Cheifetz IM. Extracorporeal membrane oxygenation for adult respiratory failure. Respir Care 2013;58(6):1038–52.
3. Firstenberg MS. Introductory chapter: evolution of ECMO from salvage to mainstream supportive and resuscitative therapy. In: Firstenberg MS, editor. Extracorporeal Membrane Oxygenation: Advances in Therapy. InTech 2016. Available at: https://www.intechopen.com/books/extracorporeal-membrane-oxygenation-advances-in-therapy/introductory-chapter-evolution-of-ecmo-from-salvage-to-mainstream-supportive-and-resuscitative-thera.
4. Tremblay L, Valenza F, Ribeiro SP, et al. Injurious ventilatory strategies increase cytokines and c-fos m-RNA expression in an isolated rat lung model. J Clin Invest 1997;99(5):944–52.
5. Schmidt M, Brechot N, Combes A. Ten situations in which ECMO is unlikely to be successful. Intensive Care Med 2016;42(5):750–2.
6. Noah MA, Peek GJ, Finney SJ, et al. Referral to an extracorporeal membrane oxygenation center and mortality among patients with severe 2009 influenza A(H1N1). JAMA 2011;306(15):1659–68.
7. Frenckner B. Extracorporeal membrane oxygenation: a breakthrough for respiratory failure. J Intern Med 2015;278(6):586–98.
8. Aokage T, Palmer K, Ichiba S, et al. Extracorporeal membrane oxygenation for acute respiratory distress syndrome. J Intensive Care 2015;3:17.
9. Munshi L, Telesnicki T, Walkey A, et al. Extracorporeal life support for acute respiratory failure. A systematic review and metaanalysis. Ann Am Thorac Soc 2014;11(5):802–10.

10. Schmidt M, Bailey M, Sheldrake J, et al. Predicting survival after extracorporeal membrane oxygenation for severe acute respiratory failure. The Respiratory Extracorporeal Membrane Oxygenation Survival Prediction (RESP) score. Am J Respir Crit Care Med 2014;189(11):1374–82.
11. Pappalardo F, Pieri M, Greco T, et al. Predicting mortality risk in patients undergoing venovenous ECMO for ARDS due to influenza A (H1N1) pneumonia: the ECMOnet score. Intensive Care Med 2013;39(2):275–81.
12. Schmidt M, Zogheib E, Roze H, et al. The PRESERVE mortality risk score and analysis of long-term outcomes after extracorporeal membrane oxygenation for severe acute respiratory distress syndrome. Intensive Care Med 2013; 39(10):1704–13.
13. Murray JF, Mattay MA, Luce J, et al. An expanded definition of the adult respiratory distress syndrome. Am Rev Respir Dis 1988;138:720–3.
14. Moerer O, Tonetti T, Quintel M. Rescue therapies for acute respiratory distress syndrome: what to try first? Curr Opin Crit Care 2017;23:8.
15. Rosenberg AA, Haft JW, Bartlett R, et al. Prolonged duration ECMO for ARDS: futility, native lung recovery, or transplantation? ASAIO J 2013;59(6):642–50.
16. Zapol WM, Snider MT, Hill JD, et al. Extracorporeal membrane oxygenation in severe acute respiratory failure. A randomized prospective study. JAMA 1979; 242(20):2193–6.
17. Terragni PP, Del Sorbo L, Mascia L, et al. Tidal volume lower than 6 ml/kg enhances lung protection role of extracorporeal carbon dioxide removal. Anesthesiology 2009;111(4):10.
18. Abrams D, Brodie D. Extracorporeal circulatory approaches to treat acute respiratory distress syndrome. Clin Chest Med 2014;35(4):765–79.
19. Webb HH, Tierney DF. Experimental pulmonary edema due to intermittent positive pressure ventilation with high inflation pressures. Protection by positive end-expiratory pressure. Am Rev Respir Dis 1974;110(5):556–65.
20. Parsons PE, Eisner MD, Thompson BT, et al. Lower tidal volume ventilation and plasma cytokine markers of inflammation in patients with acute lung injury. Crit Care Med 2005;33(1):1–6.
21. Pipeling MR, Fan E. Therapies for refractory hypoxemia in acute respiratory distress syndrome. JAMA 2010;304(22):2521–7.
22. Ranieri VM, Suter PM, Tortorella C, et al. Effect of mechanical ventilation on inflammatory mediators in patients with acute respiratory distress syndrome: a randomized controlled trial. JAMA 1999;282(1):54–61.
23. Brower RG, Lanken PN, MacIntyre N, et al. Higher versus lower positive end-expiratory pressures in patients with the acute respiratory distress syndrome. N Engl J Med 2004;351(4):327–36.
24. Gattinoni L, Tonetti T, Cressoni M, et al. Ventilator-related causes of lung injury: the mechanical power. Intensive Care Med 2016;42(10):1567–75.
25. Petrucci N, De Feo C. Lung protective ventilation strategy for the acute respiratory distress syndrome. Cochrane Database Syst Rev 2013;(2):CD003844.
26. The Acute Respiratory Distress Syndrome Network. Ventilation with lower tidal volumes as compared with traditional tidal volumes for acute lung injury and the acute respiratory distress syndrome. The Acute Respiratory Distress Syndrome Network. N Engl J Med 2000;342(18):1301–8.
27. Risnes I, Wagner K, Ueland T, et al. Interleukin-6 may predict survival in extracorporeal membrane oxygenation treatment. Perfusion 2008;23(3):173–8.
28. Mekontso Dessap A, Ware LB, Bagshaw SM. How could biomarkers of ARDS and AKI drive clinical strategies? Intensive Care Med 2016;42(5):800–2.

29. McIlwain RB, Timpa JG, Kurundkar AR, et al. Plasma concentrations of inflammatory cytokines rise rapidly during ECMO-related SIRS due to the release of preformed stores in the intestine. Lab Invest 2009;90(1):128–39.

30. von Bahr V, Hultman J, Eksborg S, et al. Long-term survival in adults treated with extracorporeal membrane oxygenation for respiratory failure and sepsis. Crit Care Med 2017;45(2):164–70.

31. Brodie D, Bacchetta M. Extracorporeal membrane oxygenation for ARDS in adults. N Engl J Med 2011;365:10.

32. Bein T, Weber-Carstens S, Goldmann A, et al. Lower tidal volume strategy (approximately 3 ml/kg) combined with extracorporeal CO2 removal versus 'conventional' protective ventilation (6 ml/kg) in severe ARDS: the prospective randomized Xtravent-study. Intensive Care Med 2013;39(5):847–56.

33. Crapo JD. Morphologic changes in pulmonary oxygen toxicity. Annu Rev Physiol 1986;48:721–31.

34. Fisher AB. Oxygen therapy. Side effects and toxicity. Am Rev Respir Dis 1980; 122(5 Pt 2):61–9.

35. Mols G, Loop T, Geiger K, et al. Extracorporeal membrane oxygenation: a ten-year experience. Am J Surg 2000;180(2):144–54.

36. Schmidt M, Pellegrino V, Combes A, et al. Mechanical ventilation during extracorporeal membrane oxygenation. Crit Care 2014;18(1):203.

37. ELSO Guidelines for Cardiopulmonary Extracorporeal Life Support. Ann Arbor (MI): Extracorporeal Life Support Organization, Version 1.3; 2013. p. 1-24. Available at: https://www.elso.org/Portals/0/IGD/Archive/FileManager/929122ae88 cusersshyerdocumentselsoguidelinesgeneralalleclsversion1.3.pdf.

38. Amato MB, Meade MO, Slutsky AS, et al. Driving pressure and survival in the acute respiratory distress syndrome. N Engl J Med 2015;372(8):747–55.

39. Serpa Neto A, Schmidt M, Azevedo LCP, et al. Associations between ventilator settings during extracorporeal membrane oxygenation for refractory hypoxemia and outcome in patients with acute respiratory distress syndrome: a pooled individual patient data analysis Mechanical ventilation during ECMO. Intensive Care Med 2016;42(11):1672–84.

40. Sutcliffe AJ. The future of ARDS. Injury 1994;25(9):587–93.

41. Cartin-Ceba R, Hubmayr RD, Qin R, et al. Predictive value of plasma biomarkers for mortality and organ failure development in patients with acute respiratory distress syndrome. J Crit Care 2015;30(1):219.e1-7.

42. Eisner MD, Thompson BT, Schoenfeld D, et al, Acute Respiratory Distress Syndrome Network. Airway pressures and early barotrauma in patients with acute lung injury and acute respiratory distress syndrome. Am J Respir Crit Care Med 2002;165(7):978–82.

43. Peek GJ, Mugford M, Tiruvoipati R, et al. Efficacy and economic assessment of conventional ventilatory support versus extracorporeal membrane oxygenation for severe adult respiratory failure (CESAR): a multicentre randomised controlled trial. Lancet 2009;374(9698):1351–63.

44. Haile DT, Schears GJ. Optimal time for initiating extracorporeal membrane oxygenation. Semin Cardiothorac Vasc Anesth 2009;13(3):146–53.

45. Kanji HD, McCallum J, Norena M, et al. Early veno-venous extracorporeal membrane oxygenation is associated with lower mortality in patients who have severe hypoxemic respiratory failure: a retrospective multicenter cohort study. J Crit Care 2016;33:169–73.

46. Sharma A, Weerwind P, Ganushchak Y, et al. Towards a proactive therapy utilizing the modern spectrum of extracorporeal life support: a single-centre experience. Perfusion 2015;30(2):113–8.

47. Kreyer S, Scaravilli V, Linden K, et al. Early utilization of extracorporeal co2 removal for treatment of acute respiratory distress syndrome due to smoke inhalation and burns in sheep. Shock 2016;45(1):65–72.

48. Wong JK, Siow VS, Hirose H, et al. End organ recovery and survival with the QuadroxD oxygenator in adults on extracorporeal membrane oxygenation. World J Cardiovasc Surg 2012;02(04):73–80.

49. Pranikoff T, Hirschl R, Steimle C, et al. Mortality is directly related to the duration of mechanical ventilation before the initiation of extracorporeal life support for severe respiratory failure. Crit Care Med 1997;25:5.

50. Kolla S, Awad SS, Rich PB, et al. Extracorporeal life support for 100 adult patients with severe respiratory failure. Ann Surg 1997;226(4):544–64 [discussion: 565–6].

51. Kahn JM, Caldwell EC, Deem S, et al. Acute lung injury in patients with subarachnoid hemorrhage: incidence, risk factors, and outcome. Crit Care Med 2006;34(1):196–202.

52. Squiers JJ, Lima B, DiMaio JM. Contemporary extracorporeal membrane oxygenation therapy in adults: fundamental principles and systematic review of the evidence. J Thorac Cardiovasc Surg 2016;152(1):20–32.

53. Patroniti N, Zangrillo A, Pappalardo F, et al. The Italian ECMO network experience during the 2009 influenza A(H1N1) pandemic: preparation for severe respiratory emergency outbreaks. Intensive Care Med 2011;37(9):1447–57.

54. Australia, New Zealand Extracorporeal Membrane Oxygenation Influenza Investigators, Davies A, Jones D, Bailey M, et al. Extracorporeal membrane oxygenation for 2009 influenza A(H1N1) acute respiratory distress syndrome. JAMA 2009;302(17):1888.

55. Hayanga AJ, Aboagye J, Esper S, et al. Extracorporeal membrane oxygenation as a bridge to lung transplantation in the United States: an evolving strategy in the management of rapidly advancing pulmonary disease. J Thorac Cardiovasc Surg 2015;149(1):291–6.

56. Shafii AE, Mason DP, Brown CR, et al. Growing experience with extracorporeal membrane oxygenation as a bridge to lung transplantation. ASAIO J 2012; 58(5):526–9.

57. Lang G, Taghavi S, Aigner C, et al. Primary lung transplantation after bridge with extracorporeal membrane oxygenation: a plea for a shift in our paradigms for indications. Transplantation 2012;93(7):729–36.

58. Hoopes CW, Kukreja J, Golden J, et al. Extracorporeal membrane oxygenation as a bridge to pulmonary transplantation. J Thorac Cardiovasc Surg 2013; 145(3):862–7 [discussion: 867–8].

59. Toyoda Y, Bhama JK, Shigemura N, et al. Efficacy of extracorporeal membrane oxygenation as a bridge to lung transplantation. J Thorac Cardiovasc Surg 2013;145(4):1065–70 [discussion: 1070–1].

60. Mason DP, Boffa DJ, Murthy SC, et al. Extended use of extracorporeal membrane oxygenation after lung transplantation. J Thorac Cardiovasc Surg 2006; 132(4):954–60.

61. Fanelli V, Costamagna A, Ranieri VM. Extracorporeal support for severe acute respiratory failure. Semin Respir Crit Care Med 2014;35(4):519–27.

62. Fuehner T, Kuehn C, Hadem J, et al. Extracorporeal membrane oxygenation in awake patients as bridge to lung transplantation. Am J Respir Crit Care Med 2012;185(7):763–8.

63. Burki NK, Mani RK, Herth FJ, et al. A novel extracorporeal CO(2) removal system: results of a pilot study of hypercapnic respiratory failure in patients with COPD. Chest 2013;143(3):678–86.

64. Braune S, Burchardi H, Engel M, et al. The use of extracorporeal carbon dioxide removal to avoid intubation in patients failing non-invasive ventilation: a cost analysis. BMC Anesthesiol 2015;15:160.

65. Gilbert CR, Vipul K, Baram M. Novel H1N1 influenza A viral infection complicated by alveolar hemorrhage. Respir Care 2010;55(5):623–5.

66. Gilbert CR, Baram M, Cavarocchi NC. "Smoking wet": respiratory failure related to smoking tainted marijuana cigarettes. Tex Heart Inst J 2013;40(1):64–7.

67. Needham DM, Yang T, Dinglas VD, et al. Timing of low tidal volume ventilation and intensive care unit mortality in acute respiratory distress syndrome. A prospective cohort study. Am J Respir Crit Care Med 2015;191(2):177–85.

68. Needham DM, Colantuoni E, Mendez-Tellez PA, et al. Lung protective mechanical ventilation and two year survival in patients with acute lung injury: prospective cohort study. BMJ 2012;344:e2124.

69. Hickling KG, Walsh J, Henderson S, et al. Low mortality rate in adult respiratory distress syndrome using low-volume, pressure-limited ventilation with permissive hypercapnia: a prospective study. Crit Care Med 1994;22:1568–78.

70. Facchin F, Fan E. Airway pressure release ventilation and high-frequency oscillatory ventilation: potential strategies to treat severe hypoxemia and prevent ventilator-induced lung injury. Respir Care 2015;60(10):1509–21.

71. Putensen C, Zech S, Wrigge H, et al. Long-term effects of spontaneous breathing during ventilatory support in patients with acute lung injury. Am J Respir Crit Care Med 2001;164(1):43–9.

72. Varpula T, Jousela I, Niemi R, et al. Combined effects of prone positioning and airway pressure release ventilation on gas exchange in patients with acute lung injury. Acta Anaesthesiol Scand 2003;47(5):516–24.

73. González M, Arroliga AC, Frutos-Vivar F, et al. Airway pressure release ventilation versus assist-control ventilation: a comparative propensity score and international cohort study. Intensive Care Med 2010;36(5):817–27.

74. Maxwell RA, Green JM, Waldrop J, et al. A randomized prospective trial of airway pressure release ventilation and low tidal volume ventilation in adult trauma patients with acute respiratory failure. J Trauma 2010;69(3):501–10 [discussion: 511].

75. Maung AA, Schuster KM, Kaplan LJ, et al. Compared to conventional ventilation, airway pressure release ventilation may increase ventilator days in trauma patients. J Trauma Acute Care Surg 2012;73(2):507–10.

76. Ferguson ND, Cook DJ, Guyatt GH, et al. High-frequency oscillation in early acute respiratory distress syndrome. N Engl J Med 2013;368(9):795–805.

77. Young D, Lamb SE, Shah S, et al. High-frequency oscillation for acute respiratory distress syndrome. N Engl J Med 2013;368(9):806–13.

78. Steinberg KP, Hudson LD, Goodman RB, et al. Efficacy and safety of corticosteroids for persistent acute respiratory distress syndrome. N Engl J Med 2006; 354(16):1671–84.

79. Ruan SY, Lin HH, Huang CT, et al. Exploring the heterogeneity of effects of corticosteroids on acute respiratory distress syndrome: a systematic review and meta-analysis. Crit Care 2014;18(2):R63.

80. Meduri GU, Golden E, Freire AX, et al. Methyprednisolone infusion in patients with early severe ARDS: results of a randomized trial. Chest 2007;131: 954–63.

81. Sibbald WJ, Short AK, Warshawski FJ, et al. Thermal dye measurements of extravascular lung water in critically ill patients. Intravascular Starling forces and extravascular lung water in the adult respiratory distress syndrome. Chest 1985;87(5):585–92.

82. National Heart Lung and, Blood Institute Acute Respiratory Distress Syndrome Clinical Trials Network, Wheeler AP, Bernard GR, Thompson BT, et al. Pulmonary-artery versus central venous catheter to guide treatment of acute lung injury. N Engl J Med 2006;354(21):2213–24.

83. Park PK. Too little oxygen: ventilation, prone positioning, and extracorporeal membrane oxygenation for severe hypoxemia. Semin Respir Crit Care Med 2016;37(1):3–15.

84. Gattinoni L, Tognoni G, Pesenti A, et al. Effect of prone positioning on the survival of patients with acute respiratory failure. N Engl J Med 2001;345(8): 568–73.

85. Taccone P, Pesenti A, Latini R, et al. Prone positioning in patients with moderate and severe acute respiratory distress syndrome: a randomized controlled trial. JAMA 2009;302(18):1977–84.

86. Guerin C, Reignier J, Richard JC, et al. Prone positioning in severe acute respiratory distress syndrome. N Engl J Med 2013;368(23):2159–68.

87. Beitler JR, Shaefi S, Montesi SB, et al. Prone positioning reduces mortality from acute respiratory distress syndrome in the low tidal volume era: a meta-analysis. Intensive Care Med 2014;40(3):332–41.

88. Sud S, Sud M, Friedrich JO, et al. Effect of mechanical ventilation in the prone position on clinical outcomes in patients with acute hypoxemic respiratory failure: a systematic review and meta-analysis. CMAJ 2008;178(9): 1153–61.

89. Searcy RJ, Morales JR, Ferreira JA, et al. The role of inhaled prostacyclin in treating acute respiratory distress syndrome. Ther Adv Respir Dis 2015;9(6): 302–12.

90. Gebistorf F, Karam O, Wetterslev J, et al. Inhaled nitric oxide for acute respiratory distress syndrome (ARDS) in children and adults. Cochrane Database Syst Rev 2016;(6):CD002787.

91. Torbic H, Szumita PM, Anger KE, et al. Inhaled epoprostenol vs inhaled nitric oxide for refractory hypoxemia in critically ill patients. J Crit Care 2013;28(5): 844–8.

92. Rose F, Zwick K, Ghofrani HA, et al. Prostacyclin enhances stretch-induced surfactant secretion in alveolar epithelial type II cells. Am J Respir Crit Care Med 1999;160(3):846–51.

93. Wen FQ, Watanabe K, Yoshida M. Inhibitory effects of interleukin-6 on release of PGI2 by cultured human pulmonary artery smooth muscle cells. Prostaglandins 1996;52(2):93–102.

94. Walmrath D, Schneider T, Schermuly R, et al. Direct comparison of inhaled nitric oxide and aerosolized prostacyclin in acute respiratory distress syndrome. Am J Respir Crit Care Med 1996;153(3):991–6.

95. Afshari A, Brok J, Moller AM, et al. Aerosolized prostacyclin for acute lung injury (ALI) and acute respiratory distress syndrome (ARDS). Cochrane Database Syst Rev 2010;(8):CD007733.

96. Dzierba AL, Abel EE, Buckley MS, et al. A review of inhaled nitric oxide and aerosolized epoprostenol in acute lung injury or acute respiratory distress syndrome. Pharmacotherapy 2014;34(3):279–90.

97. Gainnier M, Roch A, Forel JM, et al. Effect of neuromuscular blocking agents on gas exchange in patients presenting with acute respiratory distress syndrome. Crit Care Med 2004;32(1):113–9.

98. Papazian L, Forel JM, Gacouin A, et al. Neuromuscular blockers in early acute respiratory distress syndrome. N Engl J Med 2010;363(12):1107–16.

99. Alhazzani W, Alshahrani M, Jaeschke R, et al. Neuromuscular blocking agents in acute respiratory distress syndrome: a systematic review and meta-analysis of randomized controlled trials. Crit Care 2013;17(2):R43.

100. Broman LM, Holzgraefe B, Palmer K, et al. The Stockholm experience: interhospital transports on extracorporeal membrane oxygenation. Crit Care 2015; 19:278.

101. Barbaro RP, Odetola FO, Kidwell KM, et al. Association of hospital-level volume of extracorporeal membrane oxygenation cases and mortality. Analysis of the extracorporeal life support organization registry. Am J Respir Crit Care Med 2015;191(8):894–901.

102. Combes A, Brodie D, Bartlett R, et al. Position paper for the organization of extracorporeal membrane oxygenation programs for acute respiratory failure in adult patients. Am J Respir Crit Care Med 2014;190(5):488–96.

103. Lewandowski K, Rossaint R, Pappert D, et al. High survival rate in 122 ARDS patients managed according to a clinical algorithm including extracorporeal membrane oxygenation. Intensive Care Med 1997;23(8):819–35.

104. Doufle G, Roscoe A, Billia F, et al. Echocardiography for adult patients supported with extracorporeal membrane oxygenation. Crit Care 2015; 19:326.

105. Vieillard-Baron A. Is right ventricular function the one that matters in ARDS patients? Definitely yes. Intensive Care Med 2009;35(1):4–6.

106. Miranda DR, Brodie BR, Bakker J. Right ventricular unloading after initiation of venovenous extracorporeal membrane oxygenation. Am J Respir Crit Care Med 2015;191(3):346–8.

107. Vaid U, Singer E, Marhefka GD, et al. Poor positive predictive value of McConnell's sign on transthoracic echocardiography for the diagnosis of acute pulmonary embolism. Hosp Pract 2013;41(3):23–7.

108. Gray BW, Haft JW, Hirsch JC, et al. Extracorporeal life support: experience with 2,000 patients. ASAIO J 2015;61(1):2–7.

109. Maclaren G, Butt W. Extracorporeal membrane oxygenation and sepsis. Crit Care Resusc 2007;9(1):76–80.

110. Kim DW, Yeo HJ, Yoon SH, et al. Impact of bloodstream infections on catheter colonization during extracorporeal membrane oxygenation. J Artif Organs 2016;19(2):128–33.

111. Mesher A, Brogan T, Heath J, et al. ECMO-associated bloodstream infections: utility of surveillance blood cultures? Conference: 43rd Annual Critical Care Congress in Critical Care Medicine 2013. Available at: https://www.researchgate.net/publication/279018881_ECMO-associated_bloodstream_infections_Utility_of_surveillance_blood_cultures.

112. Aubron C, Cheng AC, Pilcher D, et al. Infections acquired by adults who receive extracorporeal membrane oxygenation: risk factors and outcome. Infect Control Hosp Epidemiol 2013;34(1):24–30.

113. Mateen FJ, Muralidharan R, Shinohara RT, et al. Neurological injury in adults treated with extracorporeal membrane oxygenation. Arch Neurol 2011;68(12): 1543–9.

114. Stull C, Baram M, Pitcher H, et al. Predictors of a successful wean from extracorporeal membrane oxygenation (ECMO) for acute respiratory failure syndrome (ARDS). Crit Care Med 2013;12(12):A88.

Vascular Complications in Extracoporeal Membrane Oxygenation

Kathleen M. Lamb, MD[a],*, Hitoshi Hirose, MD, PhD[b]

KEYWORDS

- Limb salvage • Venoarterial extracorporeal membrane oxygenation
- Vascular complications • Arterial dissection • Pseudoaneurysm
- Thromboembolic complications • Infectious arterial complications

KEY POINTS

- Limb ischemia is one of the most common complications of venoarterial extracorporeal membrane oxygenation (VA ECMO) via femoral cannulation.
- Use of ultrasound guidance at time of cannula placement, near infrared spectroscopy monitoring with trained intensive care unit staff during ECMO support, and placement of a distal perfusion catheter can prevent and detect early signs of limb ischemia, allowing prompt intervention.
- Other vascular complications include infection, pseudoaneurysm, dissection, retroperitoneal hematoma, and need for amputation.

INTRODUCTION

Venoarterial extracorporeal membrane oxygenation (VA ECMO) is a rescue therapy in patients with severe cardiac failure. Most patients on ECMO are cannulated via femoral artery and vein given the ready accessibility of the vessels and the emergent nature leading to need for cannulation.[1] Accessing the femoral vessels can potentially lead to significant vascular complications including limb ischemia from lack of perfusion distal to the arterial cannula, thromboembolic complications, retroperitoneal bleeding, dissection, pseudoaneurysm, and groin infection.[2–11] This article describes femoral vessel cannulation, selecting appropriate cannulas for vessel size, vascular complications associated with cannulation, and associated management strategies.

Disclosures: None for either author.
[a] Division of Vascular Surgery and Endovascular Therapy, Hospital of the University of Pennsylvania, 3400 Spruce Street, 4 Silverstein, Philadelphia, PA 19104, USA; [b] Department of Cardiothoracic Surgery, Thomas Jefferson University Hospital, 1100 Walnut Street, 5th Floor, Philadelphia, PA 19107, USA
* Corresponding author.
E-mail address: patinaras@gmail.com

We also briefly discuss venovenous ECMO (VV ECMO), which is used for respiratory support.

PATIENT EVALUATION
Vascular Access for Venoarterial Extracorporeal Membrane Oxygenation

There are 2 main cannulation strategies for patients requiring VA ECMO: central cannulation and peripheral (femoral) cannulation. VA ECMO using central cannulation is reserved for patients who are postcardiotomy with cardiac or respiratory failure. The advantage of this cannulation is simplicity of cannulation from the consequence of cardiopulmonary bypass during cardiac surgery.[12,13] The cannula size is usually larger than peripheral cannulation to provide sufficient flow to the systemic circulation. Another advantage of the central cannulation is antegrade flow to brain, compared with retrograde flow of peripheral cannulation. Cannulas are placed in direct vision of the vessels during cardiac surgery and secured with a tourniquet. Because these cannulas are a continuation of cardiopulmonary bypass, the sternum is typically kept open and packed. During an ECMO run, additional attention should be paid for cannula dislodging, mediastinal bleeding, and infections related to the open sternum.

Central cannulation is an appropriate option for patients after pericardotomy while in the operating room. Unfortunately, many of patients requiring VA ECMO present in less controlled environments than the operating room, including catherization laboratory, emergency room, intensive care unit, or the wards. In these patients, peripheral cannulation is the most appropriate option, as it can be done bedside.[1] A femoral arterial line, distal limb perfusion line, and venous line are required, and placement can be enhanced with the use of a bedside ultrasound and fluoroscopy if available. Vessel size cannot typically be assessed before the procedure with contrast imaging studies, so ultrasound findings and clinical judgment are used to estimate vessel size and guide cannula selection.[1] Small vessel size and difficulty with cannulation, including large pannus covering groin, are risk factors leading to vascular complications while placing patients on VA ECMO.[3,4,8] Distal perfusion catheters should be placed with ultrasound guidance to provide antegrade flow to the distal superficial femoral artery (SFA) and distal leg. If a vascular stent is present, cannulation from the contralateral femoral vessel is recommended to avoid damage to the stent or stent thrombosis. A previously placed inferior vena cava (IVC) filter may cause venous injury at the time of venous cannulation; thus, fluoroscopy is necessary and removal of the filter may be necessary to place the venous cannula.

Although vessels are often easily accessible, they are usually not directly visualized during cannulation, as most cannulation is done percutaneously. As such, vascular access can often be difficult, particularly in morbidly obese patients or patients with peripheral vascular disease. Given these factors, vascular complications related to VA ECMO tend to be related to peripheral femoral cannulation.[2–4] Vascular complications related to femoral cannulation are the focus of this article.

Cannula Size Selection

Each arterial and venous cannula has a flow pressure curve based on the company's package inserts. The larger cannula promises larger flow rates in the in vitro situation. For example, a 17-Fr arterial cannula is able to provide only 4 to 5 L/min, whereas a 21-Fr arterial cannula can provide 6 L/min without adding extreme pressure on the cannula, which may later lead to hemolysis. VA ECMO flow is set to achieve a goal cardiac index greater than 2.2 L/min/m^2.[14] If the cardiac distension is expected from the cardiac arrest, 1 L may be added in addition to the optimum calculated ECMO flow to decompress the heart. If the vessels are known to be small or cannulation is difficult related to small vessel caliber, a smaller cannula may be chosen to avoid catastrophic vascular injury.[1]

Vascular Access for Venovenous Extracorporeal Membrane Oxygenation

VV ECMO is reserved for isolated respiratory failure with preserved cardiac function. In VV ECMO, deoxygenated blood is drained from venous system, then passes though the ECMO circuit, and is returned to venous system. In VA ECMO, the oxygenated blood is returned to the arterial system.[15] The distribution of oxygenated blood to the patient in VV ECMO depends on the patient's own cardiac function, thus the primary indication of VV ECMO is severe acute respiratory failure (acute respiratory distress syndrome [ARDS]) despite optimum mechanical ventilation and medical treatment.[16] If cardiac function is not preserved, VV ECMO does not provide adequate oxygenation and even may lead to overdistention of the heart or pulmonary edema due to cardiac congestion.[15] Thus, preoperative evaluation of left and right ventricular function is necessary. Common contraindications for VV ECMO are those who have ventilator dependency, end-stage lung disease without a candidate for lung transplantation, and otherwise the same as VA ECMO.

The classic VV ECMO system involves bilateral femoral vein cannulation with 1 long venous cannula to the right atrium for inflow of oxygenated blood to the patient and 1 short venous cannula ending in the IVC serving as outflow of deoxygenated blood from the patient (**Fig. 1**A). Another variation of the VV ECMO system would be cannulation of the right atrium for inflow to the patient and 1 long venous cannula in the IVC from the femoral vein serving as outflow from the patient (see **Fig. 1**B). Complications of these classic VV cannulation methods include shunting of blood flow between the inflow and outflow cannulas due to the proximity of these cannulas to one another, and low flow states that occur due to IVC collapse from suction effects of the outflow cannula.

Currently, we use a double-lumen bicaval cannula (Avalon cannula, see **Fig. 1**C) for VV ECMO.[17] This cannula has 3 ports (proximal, middle, and distal). The distal port should be located in the IVC to drain deoxygenated blood from the lower extremities, and the proximal port is located in the superior vena cava to drain the upper extremities. The middle port is placed in the right atrium facing the tricuspid valve to allow oxygenated blood from the pump to be delivered to the patient. This cannula design minimizes the inflow-outflow reperfusion or shunting. Because of this particular positioning of the ports, cannulation should be performed under fluoroscopy and confirmed with echocardiography. Other advantages of the Avalon cannula are (1) single cannulation, (2) minimizing shunting or recirculation, and (3) avoidance of femoral cannulation. Because the Avalon cannulation does not require femoral cannulation, proning of the patient would be relatively easy, which is a relatively common intervention to improve oxygenation and lung recruitment for patients with ARDS. Avoiding a femoral cannulation also allows patients to sit up in bed or even ambulate while on VV ECMO support. Limitations of the Avalon cannula are its ridged design and that it only affords placement via the right internal jugular vein (RIJV).

Care must be taken during placement of the Avalon cannula via the RIJV to prevent wire or cannula migration into or through the right ventricle. Using fluoroscopy, the guidewire can carefully be directed into the IVC. Ensuring cannula position in the IVC prevents inadvertent migration of the cannula into the right ventricle, preventing adequate oxygenation to occur, or right ventricle perforation by the cannula resulting in cardiac tamponade.[18] Another potential issue is cannula rotation during ECMO run. If the outflow is not appropriately facing the tricuspid valve, the oxygenated blood may

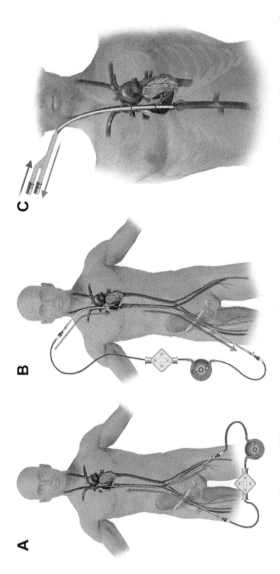

Fig. 1. (*A*) Classic VV ECMO cannulation with long venous cannula in right atrium and shorter cannula in the IVC. (*B*) A variation of ECMO cannulation with cannulation of the right atrium and a long venous cannula in the IVC. (*C*) Double-lumen bicaval cannula (Avalon cannula) for VV ECMO inserted into the RIJV.

not circulate effectively. If the oxygenation by VV ECMO is not adequate, radiograph, fluoroscopy, or echocardiogram can be used to confirm the Avalon position.[15]

VASCULAR COMPLICATIONS

Due to the large cannula (15–24-Fr) sizes needed to provide life-sustaining oxygenated circulation through the ECMO circuit, vascular complications can prove to be a clinical challenge in treating these patients. As a result, acute and late limb ischemia has been reported to be on the order of 10% to 70%.[2–9] Other complications that may arise from placement of cannulas include dissection, pseudoaneurysm formation, groin infection, and retroperitoneal bleeding. Appropriate prevention and treatment of vascular limb complications is imperative, particularly as limb ischemia is associated with decreased survival to hospital discharge.[19] This section discusses complications and focuses on management strategies.

Thromboembolic Complications

Clinical manifestations
Thromboembolic complications are responsible for most limb complications associated with femoral arterial cannulation. As mentioned, given the large size of femoral cannulas, placement in femoral arteries can be occlusive or near occlusive, obstructing flow distal to perfuse the leg. Patients particularly at risk include those with peripheral arterial disease, women, who traditionally have smaller vessel diameter than men, and young patients who have not yet developed collateral circulation that comes with progressive atherosclerosis with age.[1,2,8,9] Additionally, difficult cannulation was predictive of future limb ischemia while on VA ECMO.[1,2,4,8,9] Diagnosis of acute limb ischemia includes physical examination demonstrating ischemia, including pain, pallor, poikilothermia, gangrene, motor or sensor deficit, and loss of pedal Doppler signals. If not able to be appropriately managed, ischemia will persist, and limb loss may be inevitable. Rhabdomyolysis due to limb ischemia may lead into acute renal failure and can result in life-threating complications. Additionally, thromboembolic complications can occur related to stasis of blood in the cannulated limb (arterial or venous) or distal embolization. Therapeutic anticoagulation during cannulation, and while on the VA ECMO circuit, may help prevent ischemia.

Treatment of ischemic complications
As limb ischemia is the most significant complication of VA ECMO cannulation, much research has been done to investigate strategies to prevent and treat ongoing limb ischemia. Placement of a distal arterial perfusion catheter (DPC) has been demonstrated in all series to prevent or reverse the effects of limb ischemia after cannulation in both adult[2–4,8–10,20–22] and pediatric patients.[23–25] The distal perfusion catheter (4-Fr or 5-Fr catheter) is placed using an 0.018-inch micropuncture wire (Cook Medical, Bloomington, IN) antegrade into the SFA under ultrasound guidance and attached to a 3-way stopcock of the side port of the ipsilateral arterial cannula. This catheter removes blood from the retrograde arterial cannula and allows antegrade perfusion into the SFA (**Fig. 2**). We advocate DPC placement at the time of cannulation if feasible.[1,8] Additionally, heparin (5000mg bolus with weight based infusion) (or argatroban [0.2mcg/kg/min in patients with normal hepatic function] in the situation of heparin-induced thrombocytopenia), used to prevent thrombosis of the ECMO circuit,[8] also reduces the incidence of limb ischemia.

Some have described use of a distal venous drainage line attached to the side port of the venous cannula to allow drainage of the leg in situations in which the femoral venous cannula was occlusive.[26–28] Although venous hypertension after placement

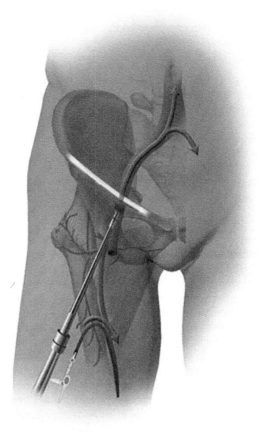

Fig. 2. Illustration of femoral arterial cannulation with distal perfusion catheter. Flow is retrograde into the iliac artery with antegrade flow from the femoral cannula to the SFA via distal perfusion catheter to perfuse the leg.

of the venous cannula has not been as well described, venous stasis leading to leg edema after cannula placement is well known and may exacerbate limb ischemia. Russo and colleagues[26] advocate for placement of a venous drainage cannula in addition to an arterial DPC to allow venous drainage from the limb. Distal drainage cannulas are a small caliber (similar to DPC, 5 Fr) and are at risk for thrombosis, although patency can be maintained with routine flushing of the line with heparin.

Additional methods to prevent limb ischemia include use of near infrared spectroscopy (NIRS) in addition to vigilant physical examination by trained intensive care staff. NIRS pads are placed immediately after cannulation onto the legs to provide baseline values for limb perfusion.[8,29–34] Baseline NIRS of peripheral capillary oxygen saturation (SpO_2) greater than 40 to 50 has been demonstrated in the literature to correlate with good limb perfusion.[32,33] Any decline in baseline NIRS or NIRS SpO_2 less than 40 suggests limb ischemia and should prompt further investigation.[2,30,31] If NIRS declines, Doppler signals should be checked and if present, NIRS pads or monitors should be changed and the patient reevaluated. If there is a loss of Doppler signals, the distal perfusion catheter can be investigated and placed if previously absent or replaced if thrombosis is suspected.[8]

Limb revascularization with a distal perfusion catheter after acute limb ischemia may lead to reperfusion injury, including lower extremity compartment syndrome. Clinical manifestations of compartment syndrome include edematous, tense calf or thigh, pain, paresthesias, paralysis, or inability to dorsiflex the foot and, often, vascular congestion of the digits. Prompt recognition of compartment syndrome is necessary and requires 4-compartment fasciotomies to release excessive intracompartmental pressure leading to limb ischemia and neurologic compromise of the leg. If ECMO is ongoing at the time of fasciotomies, anticoagulation may need to be adjusted to prevent ongoing bleeding complications. Alternatively, unrecognized or untreated limb ischemia may lead to gangrene and tissue loss, ultimately requiring amputation. Additionally, monitoring must be ongoing for rhabdomyolysis after limb reperfusion, including monitoring of creatine phosphokinase, urine myoglobin, and potassium. Patients experiencing rhabdomyolysis may have tea-colored urine and require ongoing hydration (**Fig. 3**).

At the time of decannulation, open repair of the femoral arteriotomy, with or without patch angioplasty, can prevent arterial stenosis and further complications of peripheral arterial occlusive disease or acute limb ischemia.[2,4,8,10] Femoral venous access can be closed using a purse-string. We perform decannulation in the operating

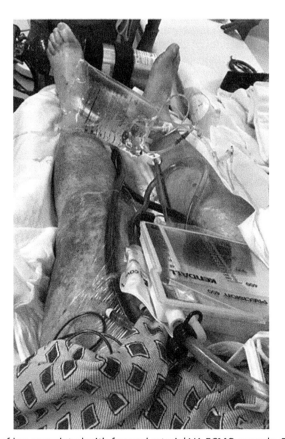

Fig. 3. Ischemia of leg cannulated with femoral arterial VA ECMO cannula. Foley containing tea-colored urine indicative of rhabdomyolysis.

room with approximately 1 hour of operative time. Arterial patch angioplasty may make arterial decannulation difficult, but it could be done via femoral cutdown in the operative room or access can be obtained via the contralateral femoral artery. If thromboembolic complications occur at the time of decannulation or in the perioperative period, a thrombectomy can be performed. Limb ischemia after decannulation may occur related to arterial stenosis from preexisting peripheral arterial disease or related to arterial stenosis from arteriotomy closure. In these circumstances, endovascular methods, including balloon angioplasty or stenting can be performed. Additionally, open reconstruction of the femoral vessels with endarterectomy and patch angioplasty or femoral-femoral bypass grafting can improve arterial inflow.[4] In patients with irrecoverable limb ischemia, amputation may be necessary, with reported rates of up to 14% of patients with limb ischemia.[2–4,8,10,20]

Our institutional experience has led us to advocate for use of a protocol to approach patients on VA ECMO to prevent limb ischemia, including the methods described previously. We place DPC at the time of arterial cannulation, unless extenuating circumstances prevent. In situations when DPC is not placed at cannulation, it is placed in the intensive care unit (ICU) when the patient stabilizes or if ischemic symptoms develop. Additionally, all patients have NIRS monitoring placed immediately to obtain baseline perfusion values and then these numbers are trended in an effort to identify a change in limb perfusion before clinical manifestations. Additionally, ICU nursing, physician extenders, and physicians are all trained to perform appropriate physical examinations on these patients to identify limb ischemia early. At the time of decannulation, we perform open repair of the femoral artery with patch angioplasty (using a patch to close the arteriotomy) to prevent arterial stenosis and further limb ischemia.[8] Following this strict protocol, we have been able to successfully salvage limbs cannulated for VA ECMO without the need for amputation and preserve use of a functional limb.

Vessel Damage

Clinical manifestations
In addition to ischemia, other vascular complications may occur at the time of cannulation, including pseudoaneurysm formation, dissection, and development of a retroperitoneal bleed. Pseudoaneurysm is reported in the literature to occur in up to 14%,[9] dissection in 7% to 14%,[3,9] and retroperitoneal hematoma has been reported in only 1 study in 1 of 15 patients (7%).[9] These complications typically occur at the time of cannulation, with increased risk when cannulation is difficult.[4]

Clinical manifestations of pseudoaneurysm can include bruising of the effected groin, a palpable bulge, or new thigh numbness. Presentation of dissection can be variable; from asymptomatic to absence of flow after starting the ECMO circuit, but should be on the differential if limb ischemia presents. Retroperitoneal bleed may present with flank pain and a decline in hemoglobin, which often can be associated with oliguria; all signs of bleeding. Computerized tomographic arteriography is the gold standard imaging test to evaluate all of these complications.[35]

Prevention and treatment
Access site complications (pseudoaneurysm, dissection, and retroperitoneal bleed) can potentially be minimized. Careful cannula placement using ultrasound guidance is the gold standard when accessing femoral vessels percutaneously to prevent a high arterial stick or arteriotomy in a location unable to be compressed on the femoral head.[35]

Once diagnosis of pseudoaneurysm, dissection, or retroperitoneal bleed is made, conservative management or surgical intervention needs to be decided.

Pseudoaneurysms at the cannula site can be repaired at the time of decannulation with an open arteriotomy repair. Dissections can be either watched conservatively, or stented in the event of a flow limiting dissection leading to limb ischemia. In the event that the dissection is symptomatic and VA ECMO is still needed, a new arterial cannula can be placed into the contralateral femoral artery. Retroperitoneal bleeds can be either monitored if small and the patient is hemodynamically stable, or washed out via a retroperitoneal incision with drain placement. Decision regarding continued anticoagulation while on VA ECMO with a retroperitoneal bleed needs to be made with options of discontinuing the drip, or continuing at a low therapeutic goal in the event of a stable hemoglobin. Patients may need to be transfused if signs of bleeding persist.[36]

Infection

Clinical manifestations

Femoral cannulation for VA ECMO can be complicated by superficial groin or deep space arterial infection given the location of cannulas in the groin. Infection rates have been reported as 7% to 20% in the VA ECMO population.[3,4,8,9] Wound infections can be further complicated in the morbidly obese or malnourished. Soft tissue groin infections may manifest as cellulitis, induration, or drainage from around the cannulas or through a decannulated and closed groin. Patients may have systemic signs, including fevers, hypotension, leukocytosis, and bacteremia. Similarly, patients may develop deep space or arterial infections related to systemic bacteremia or progression of a superficial wound infection. Infected wounds can lead to significant morbidity and mortality, particularly when associated with gram-negative organisms.[37–39] Early recognition of infection can lead to early treatment before development of systemic sepsis.

Prevention and treatment of infection

Groin infections after VA ECMO cannulation can be prevented with the use of sterile technique during cannula placement and use of periprocedural antibiotics. Once an infection is identified, antibiotics should be initiated early, and the need for surgical treatment should be determined. If there is concerning drainage from a wound, wide local debridement should be performed and decannulation if feasible. Wounds can be left open with wet to dry packing. Once gross infection has been cleared, a negative-pressure wound dressing can accelerate wound healing in our experience.[8] If femoral vessels are exposed, soft tissue coverage must be provided either by closure of deep tissue or mobilization of a local muscle flap, usually sartorius or gracilis muscle.[37,40]

SUMMARY

Emergent femoral cannulation for VA ECMO can lead to profound vascular complications predominately related to limb ischemia. A comprehensive protocol to prevent, monitor, and treat limb ischemia when present is imperative and results in successful limb salvage.[8] Cannula placement with ultrasound guidance and an ICU team trained to monitor limbs for signs of ischemia is necessary. Adjunctively, NIRS limb monitoring may be able to detect ischemia before it becomes clinically apparent, and distal perfusion catheter placement is imperative to provide antegrade limb perfusion with an often near-occlusive cannula in the common femoral artery. Beyond this, ongoing limb ischemia may require anticoagulation and surgical intervention to allow salvage of an ischemic limb.

REFERENCES

1. Lamb KM, Hirose H, Cavarocchi NC. Preparation and technical considerations for percutaneous cannulation for veno-arterial extracorporeal membrane oxygenation. J Card Surg 2013;28:190–2.
2. Foley PJ, Morris RJ, Woo EY, et al. Limb ischemia during femoral cannulation for cardiopulmonary support. J Vasc Surg 2010;52:850–3.
3. Bisdas T, Beutel G, Warnecke G, et al. Vascular complications in patients undergoing femoral cannulation for extracorporeal membrane oxygenation support. Ann Thorac Surg 2011;92:626–31.
4. Zimpfer D, Heinisch B, Czerny M, et al. Late vascular complications after extracorporeal membrane oxygenation support. Ann Thorac Surg 2006;81:892–5.
5. D'Alessandro C, Aubert S, Golmard JL, et al. Extracorporeal membrane oxygenation temporary support for early graft failure after cardiac transplantation. Eur J Cardiothorac Surg 2010;37:343–9.
6. Pranikoff T, Hirschl RB, Remenapp R, et al. Venovenous extracorporeal life support via percutaneous cannulation in 94 patients. Chest 1999;3:818–22.
7. Avalli L, Sangalli F, Migliari M, et al. Early vascular complications after percutaneous cannulation for extracorporeal membrane oxygenation for cardiac assist. Minerva Anestesiol 2016;82(1):36–43.
8. Lamb KM, DiMuzio PJ, Johnson A, et al. Arterial protocol including prophylactic distal perfusion catheter decreases limb ischemia complications in patients undergoing extracorporeal membrane oxygenation. J Vasc Surg 2017;65(4): 1074–9.
9. Roussel A, Al-Attar N, Alkhoder S, et al. Outcomes of percutaneous femoral cannulation for venoarterial extracorporeal membrane oxygenation support. Eur Heart J Acute Cardiovasc Care 2012;1(2):111–4.
10. Vallabhajosyula P, Kramer M, Lazar S, et al. Lower-extremity complications with femoral extracorporeal life support. J Thorac Cardiovasc Surg 2016;15:1738–44.
11. Aziz F, Brehm CE, El-Banyosy A, et al. Arterial complications in patients undergoing extracorporeal membrane oxygenation via femoral cannulation. Ann Vasc Surg 2014;28:178–82.
12. Jayaraman AL, Cormican D, Shah P, et al. Cannulation strategies in adult veno-arterial and veno-venous extracorporeal membrane oxygenation: techniques, limitations, and special considerations. Ann Card Anaesth 2017;20(Suppl): S11–8.
13. Reeb J, Olland A, Renaud S, et al. Vascular access for extracorporeal life support: tips and tricks. J Thorac Dis 2016;8:S353–63.
14. Unai S, Nguyen M, Tanaka D, et al. Clinical significance of spontaneous echo contrast on extracorporeal membrane oxygenation. Ann Thorac Surg 2017; 103(3):773–8.
15. Shaheen A, Tanaka D, Cavarocchi NC, et al. Veno-venous extracorporeal membrane oxygenation (VV ECMO) indications, preprocedural considerations, and technique. J Card Surg 2016;31:248–52.
16. Brodie D, Bacchetta M. Extracorporeal membrane oxygenation for ARDS in adults. N Engl J Med 2011;365:1905–14.
17. Javidfar J, Brodie D, Wang D. Use of bicaval dual-lumen catheter for adult venovenous extracorporeal membrane oxygenation. Ann Thorac Surg 2011;91: 1763–8.

18. Hirose H, Yamane K, Marhefka G, et al. Right ventricular rupture and tamponade caused by malposition of the Avalon cannula for venovenous extracorporeal membrane oxygenation. J Cardiothorac Surg 2012;7:36.
19. Tanaka D, Hirose H, Cavarocchi NC, et al. The impact of vascular complications on survival of patients on venoarterial extracorporeal membrane circulation. Ann Thorac Surg 2016;101:1729–34.
20. Muehrcke DD, McCarthy PM, Stewart RW, et al. Complications of extracorporeal life support systems using heparin-bonded surfaces: the risk of intracardiac clot formation. J Thorac Cardiovasc Surg 1995;110:843–51.
21. Madershahian N, Nagib R, Wippermann J, et al. A simple technique of distal limb perfusion during prolonged femoro-femoral cannulation. J Card Surg 2006;21:168–9.
22. Greason KL, Hemp JR, Maxwell M, et al. Prevention of distal limb ischemia during cardiopulmonary support via femoral cannulation. Ann Thorac Surg 1995;60:209–10.
23. Gander JW, Fisher JC, Reichstein AR, et al. Limb ischemia after common femoral artery cannulation for venoarterial extracorporeal membrane oxygenation: an unresolved problem. J Pediatr Surg 2010;45:2136–40.
24. Haley MJ, Fisher JC, Ruiz-Elizalde AR, et al. Percutaneous distal perfusion of the lower extremity after femoral cannulation for venoarterial extracorporeal membrane oxygenation in a small child. J Ped Surg 2009;44:437–40.
25. Schad CA, Fallow BP, Monteagudo J, et al. Routine use of distal perfusion in pediatric femoral venoarterial extracorporeal membrane oxygenation. Artif Organs 2017;41(1):11–6.
26. Russo CF, Cannata A, Vitali E, et al. Prevention of limb ischemia and edema during peripheral venoarterial extracorporeal membrane oxygenation in adults. J Card Surg 2009;24:185–7.
27. DiBella I, Enrico R, Da UC, et al. Is lower limb venous drainage during peripheral extracorporeal membrane oxygenation necessary? ASAIO J 2010;56(1):35–6.
28. LeGuyader A, Lacroix P, Ferrat P, et al. Venous leg congestion treated with distal venous drainage during peripheral extracorporeal membrane oxygenation. Artif Organs 2006;30(8):633–4.
29. Wong JK, Smith TN, Pitcher HT, et al. Cerebral and lower limb near-infrared spectroscopy in adults on extracorporeal membrane oxygenation. Artif Organs 2012;36(8):659–67.
30. Huang SC, Yu Y, Ko WJ, et al. Pressure criterion for placement of distal perfusion catheter to prevent limb ischemia during adult extracorporeal life support. J Thorac Cardiovasc Surg 2004;128:776–7.
31. Schachner T, Bonaros N, Bonatti J, et al. Near infrared spectroscopy for controlling the quality of distal leg perfusion in remote access cardiopulmonary bypass. Eur J Cardiothorac Surg 2008;34:1253–4.
32. Yao F, Tseng C, Ho C, et al. Cerebral oxygenation is associated with early postoperative neuropsychological dysfunction in patients undergoing cardiac surgery. J Cardiothorac Vasc Anesth 2004;18(5):552–8.
33. Steffen RJ, Sale S, Anandamurthy B, et al. Using near-infared spectroscopy tp monitor lower extremities in patients on venoarterial extracorporeal membrane oxygenation. Ann Thorac Surg 2014;95(5):1853–4.
34. Kim DJ, Cho YJ, Park SH, et al. Near-infrared spectroscopy monitoring for early detection of limb ischemia in patients on veno-arterial extracorporeal membrane oxygenation. ASAIO J 2017. [Epub ahead of print].

35. Sambol EB, Mckinsey JF. Local complications: endovascular. In: Cronenwett JL, Johnson W, editors. Rutherford's vascular surgery. 8th edition. Philadelphia: Elsevier; 2014. p. 704–22.

36. Turney EJ, Lydon SP. Technique: endovascular diagnostic. In: Cronenwett JL, Johnson W, editors. Rutherford's vascular surgery. 8th edition. Philadelphia: Elsevier; 2014. p. 1304–21.

37. Kalish A, Farber A, Homa K, et al. Factors associated with surgical site infection after lower extremity bypass in the Society for Vascular Surgery (SVS) Vascular Quality Initiative (VQI). J Vasc Surg 2014;60(5):1238–46.

38. Leon RJ, Thai J, Pacanowski JP. Gram-negative groin sepsis treated with covered stents and systemic antibiotics. Vascular 2011;4:226–31.

39. Patrut GV, Neamtu C, Ionac M. Leg for life? The use of Sartorius muscle flap for the treatment of an infected vascular reconstructions after VA-ECMO use. A case report. Int J Surg Case Rep 2015;16:25–8.

40. Shih PK, Cheng HT, Wu CI, et al. Management of infected groin wounds after vascular surgery. Surg Infect (Larchmt) 2013;14(3):325–30.

Pediatric Extracorporeal Membrane Oxygenation

Christopher Loren Jenks, MD[a], Lakshmi Raman, MD[b], Heidi J. Dalton, MD[c,d],*

KEYWORDS

- Pediatric extracorporeal membrane oxygenation
- Pediatric extracorporeal life support • Centrifugal technology • Fluid overload
- Nutrition

KEY POINTS

- Pediatric extracorporeal membrane oxygenation (ECMO) is a growing field.
- Many centers started with roller pumps but have transitioned to centrifugal pumps.
- Modes of support include venovenous for respiratory support and venoarterial for cardiac support.
- Diuretics, slow continuous ultrafiltration, and continuous renal replacement can be used to manage fluid overload.
- Provide adequate nutrition, preferably use the enteral route if possible.

INTRODUCTION

Extracorporeal life support (ECLS), commonly referred to as extracorporeal membrane oxygenation (ECMO), is a modified form of cardiopulmonary bypass. Venous blood is drained from the patient and advanced to a membrane lung for gas exchange. Oxygenated blood is then returned to the patient through a large vein (called venovenous or VV ECMO) or artery (called venoarterial or VA ECMO). Although ECMO was attempted early on in adults, failure to demonstrate any benefit cooled any enthusiasm for the technique, and it was largely abandoned for adults until recently. Experience in ECMO has come largely from the neonatal and pediatric population.

Disclosure Statement: Dr H.J. Dalton discloses that she is a consultant for Innovative ECMO Concepts Inc, rEVO biologics and has provided speaker support for Maquet Inc.
[a] Department of Pediatrics, Section Critical Care Medicine, Cardiac Intensive Care Unit, Baylor College of Medicine, Texas Children's Hospital, 6621 Fannin Street, Houston, TX 77030, USA; [b] Department of Pediatrics, Section Critical Care Medicine, University of Texas Southwestern Medical Center at Dallas, Children's Medical Center at Dallas, 5323 Harry Hines Boulevard, Dallas, TX 75390, USA; [c] Department of Pediatrics, Adult and Pediatric ECMO, INOVA Fairfax Medical Center, Inova Fairfax Hospital, 3300 Gallows Road, Falls Church, VA 22042, USA; [d] George Washington University, 2121 I Street Northwest, Washington, DC 20052, USA
* Corresponding author. Inova Fairfax Hospital, 3300 Gallows Road, Falls Church, VA 22042.
E-mail address: Heidi.dalton26@gmail.com

Crit Care Clin 33 (2017) 825–841
http://dx.doi.org/10.1016/j.ccc.2017.06.005
0749-0704/17/© 2017 Elsevier Inc. All rights reserved.

In 1975, the work of Robert Bartlett and colleagues propelled ECMO forward by supporting the first neonate with persistent pulmonary hypertension.[1] After this initial experience, others also pioneered ECMO support in infants. Although premature infants had a high incidence of intracranial hemorrhage, term infants did well. Several randomized trials in the United States and the United Kingdom found that ECMO support improved outcomes when compared with conventional care[2] and it has become accepted practice in neonatal care.

As experience with neonatal ECMO grew, application to children outside the infant period began to expand. Most information on the use of ECMO comes from the Extracorporeal Life Support Organization (ELSO) international registry. Of the more than 80,000 patients reported, more than 8000 pediatric patients with respiratory failure have received ECMO support and 9300 have been supported for cardiac dysfunction. **Table 1** outlines outcomes based on diagnosis from the ELSO registry. All centers should report data to ELSO and follow center-specific reports for quality improvement and benchmarking. Recent advancements in technology have been associated with expansion to more complex patient populations. The following will describe current technology, management complications, and future needs of these critically ill children.

EQUIPMENT AND EXTRACORPOREAL MODES
Circuit

Blood is drained from the patient to a pump that advances blood to a membrane lung. Gas exchange, which removes carbon dioxide and adds oxygen to the blood, occurs and the oxygenated return is directed back into the patient via a large cannula placed in a vein or artery. As membrane lungs have become very low resistance and efficient, ECMO also can be performed in some circumstances without need for a pump. In this circumstance (pumpless ECMO), the patient's native blood pressure drives blood from an arterial source through the circuit and membrane lung and back in to the venous circulation. This mode also can be used in patients with severe pulmonary hypertension, as pressure from the right ventricle can drive blood through a cannula placed in the pulmonary artery to the membrane lung and oxygenated return directed into the left side of the heart or the aorta. Conversely, if a patient has adequate pulmonary function and just needs circulatory support, the membrane lung can be omitted and the ECMO circuit used for hemodynamic support.

Roller Pumps

In the early days of ECMO, most centers used a roller head located with an enclosed box termed "pump housing."[3] Roller pumps advance blood through the circuit tubing

Table 1					
ECLS registry report: January 2017					
		Survived ECLS		Survived to DC or Transfer	
Pediatric	Total Patients	Total Number	Percentage	Total Number	Percentage
Respiratory	8070	5424	67	4632	57
Cardiac	9362	6404	68	4758	50
ECPR	3399	1958	57	1414	41

Abbreviations: DC, discharge; ECLS, extracorporeal life support; ECPR, extracorporeal cardiopulmonary resuscitation.

to a steel roller that rotates and compresses the blood against the wall of the pump housing. Blood exits the pump head at high pressure and is advanced to the membrane lung where gas exchange occurs. After the blood is oxygenated, it is then returned to the patient. The roller pump is dependent on gravity drainage to maintain preload.[3] Roller pumps generate high pressure in the circuit distal to the tubing/pump housing. Any acute interruption to forward flow, as may occur with kinking of the arterial cannula or any obstruction to forward flow on the high-pressure side of the circuit, can result in immediate and potentially lethal circuit rupture. Monitoring of the high-pressure side of the ECMO circuit is universal, with critical high limits for arterial line pressure determined based on tubing size and pump flow. Pressures lower than 300 to 350 mm Hg are desired, and safety mechanisms will stop the ECMO pump if line pressure limits are exceeded. Proper setting of occlusion of tubing against the pump housing is also important, as too loose occlusion can lead to inadequate forward flow, whereas too tight occlusion can lead to stress on the tubing within the pump housing and rupture. Periodic rotation of the tubing within the pump housing requires an increased length of tubing within the circuit and makes priming volume of roller head circuits greater than that with centrifugal devices. Although centrifugal pumps have replaced roller-head devices in many institutions and are used almost universally for adult ECMO, roller systems remain fairly common in neonatal and pediatric sites. Long experience and familiarity with them, and concerns over potential increased hemolysis from low flows in centrifugal pumps, are potential benefits. Disadvantages include the need for long circuit lengths to augment gravity venous drainage and the need to periodically rotate the tubing with the pump housing. They are also harder to move around on transport, as their large motor and associated circuitry gives them a large "footprint." In a survey from 2011, 85% of neonatal centers used roller-pump devices. A recent study of patients younger than 19 years between 2012 and 2014 noted that centrifugal pumps were used 65% of the time.

Centrifugal Pumps

Technological improvements and the arrival of low-resistance oxygenators have resulted in the transition to centrifugal pump systems. Although older models were plagued with hemolysis at low flows that infants and children require, newer devices now use small pump-heads that may be magnetically levitated or function via bearings that are low resistance, extremely durable, and create less heat, which may lessen risk of hemolysis. The high resistance within silicone membrane oxygenator also made it difficult for centrifugal devices to push blood through the device without inducing hemolysis. Although centrifugal pumps generate high negative pressure on the venous inflow side, forward flow is created only if downstream pressure is lower than the pressure in the pump head. Thus, occlusion of the post–centrifugal pump circuit will not generate high pressures such as can occur in roller head devices and tubing rupture risk is low. Rotation of either roller head or centrifugal pumps results in generation of high negative pressure in the ECMO tubing that can lead to hemolysis and cavitation as air is drawn out of solution. The collapse of the tubing and cannula that can be induced by high negative pressure also can lead to damage of the endothelium of the affected vessel or the right atrium. It is also postulated that, as clots develop in the membrane oxygenator over time and increase outflow resistance, hemolysis worsens in the rotor head. Centrifugal pumps also may create micro-emboli that can reach the patient if they are not trapped in the membrane lung. New low-resistance hollow-fiber membrane lungs allow easy propulsion of blood from the centrifugal device, and are a major reason that centrifugal pumps have become so popular for patients of all ages.

Pressure and Flow Monitors

Although any access sites into the circuit pose a risk for air embolus (if on the venous side) or rapid bleeding from open stopcocks (if on the arterial side), most centers will maintain some sites for safety monitoring to prevent excessive negative pressure or high pressure on the post pump side. The pressure difference across the oxygenator, the amount of negative pressure applied to the patient (inlet or suction pressure), flow to the patient (outlet or line pressure), and flow through any type of shunt placed within the circuit are typical monitoring sites. Higher negative pressures (inlet pressure) can cause damage to the heart valves, and cause cavitation resulting in hemolysis.[4] Higher outlet (line pressure) may result from systemic hypertension, high flow into a small cannula (high resistance) or kinking or obstruction to the outlet side of the circuit. Any lack of forward flow exposes red cells in the pump head to increased shear stress and may result in severe hemolysis. Many of newer pump systems incorporate pressure and flow monitoring into their systems.[4]

Membrane Lungs

Initially, centers used silicone membrane lungs, which are efficient in gas exchange, but have high resistance to blood flow entering the device. As new, low-resistance membrane lungs have been developed, use of the silicone membrane has almost disappeared in ECMO centers.[3] The design of the hollow-fiber oxygenator allows blood to flow through one side of the membrane, and a counter-current stream of oxygenated gas to flow on the other side of the membrane. The key factors determining oxygen exchange within the oxygenator are the following: type of oxygenator and diffusion characteristics or coefficients, surface area of membrane, viscosity of the blood, ECMO blood flow rate, and the fractional inspired oxygen (Fio_2).[3]

Membrane lungs come in different sizes with varying blood flow and gas exchange rates. Selecting the optimal oxygenator for the patient is an important part of circuit design. If a large membrane lung is used in a small patient, the required patient flow may be lower than that recommended by the manufacturer for the device. Some centers will merely ignore this fact and watch for clotting or malfunction in the device. Some centers will run a shunt line around the oxygenator, which keeps the flow through the device above the minimal suggested rate. As smaller-membrane lungs have become available, more choices now exist to match expected flow rates and membrane lung size. Increased complications have been observed when changing to new oxygenators and every center must develop appropriate training and evaluation regimens when introducing new equipment.[5]

The optimal flow is provided by a cannula with a short length and large diameter (remember the Poiseuille Law). Different manufacturers have different specifications (rated ECMO flows) for the different size cannulas (**Table 2**). Ideally, one should try to select a cannula that will provide the expected ECMO flow at a pressure drop of less than 100 mm Hg.[3] A pressure drop greater than 100 mm Hg can be a significant factor in the development of hemolysis.[3] Pressure drops for various cannulas are often provided by manufacturers, although studies are done with water and not blood. Other work has noted that negative pressure of greater than −20 results in endothelial damage within the right atrium. Thus, if a venous pressure alarm is used, the set point is optimally 20 mm Hg lower than the pressure drop across the cannula. Tubing sizes come in one-quarter, one-half, and three-eighths inch. When selecting a circuit for a small patient, matching tubing size to cannula connectors is important to consider during setup and initiation.

Table 2
Rated cannula flows in milliliters

Manufacturer Size, Fr	Venous	Arterial	Double-Lumen: Origen (Biomedical, Austin, TX)	Double-Lumen: Avalon (MAQUET Holding BV & Co, Rastatt, Germany)
8	500	500	—	—
10	900	900	—	—
12	1500	1500	—	—
13	—	—	410	740
14	2600	2400	—	—
15	1300	—	—	—
16	—	—	675	675
17	1900	3600	—	—
18	—	—	—	—
19	2600	3800	920	920
21	3200	5000	—	—
23	5000	—	2000	2000
25	6000	—	—	—
27	6500	—	—	—
28	—	—	3000	—
31	—	—	—	5000
32	—	—	5000	—

Modes of Support: Venovenous Support

Multiple studies demonstrate that VV support is associated with fewer neurologic complications and better outcome when compared with VA support. Severity of illness information is often not available for these reports, and it is unclear if outcome is improved because the patients are "less sick." Potential advantages of VV support include oxygenated return into the pulmonary circuit, which may decrease hypoxia-induced pulmonary vascular resistance; debris returning from the circuit being trapped in lungs rather than the arterial system; and avoidance of artery cannulation. VV support is used in most adult respiratory patients receiving ECMO, and has gained traction in neonates and children as well. VV support in neonates is approximately 25% and 50% in pediatric patients according to the latest ELSO registry report (January 2017). Traditionally, neonatal and pediatric VV support was via double-lumen cannulas placed in the right internal jugular vein. As drainage and return are both within a few millimeters of each other, recirculation of oxygenated blood is a disadvantage of these devices. More recently, a double-lumen cannula (Avalon, MAQUET Holding BV & Co, Rastatt, Germany) with drainage from both the superior vena cava and inferior vena cava (IVC) and return directed to the tricuspid valve when placed correctly, has become popular. It is difficult to place without fluoroscopy and movement of the IVC portion into the hepatic vessels or back into the right atrium is a problem especially in small children. The 13-Fr Avalon has been redesigned without the IVC drainage site due to reports of cardiac perforation. Femoral vessels are not of adequate size for venous drainage or arterial return until approximately 15 kg or 2 years of age. As many children are receiving vasoactive infusions before ECMO, concerns over adequacy of cardiac function often lead clinicians to choose VA support as the initial mode. Studies in children have noted, however, that once adequate oxygenation is applied with VV ECMO and high pressures from mechanical ventilation reduced, need for vasoactive medications often disappears.[6]

Modes of Support: Venoarterial Support

VA support provides the most oxygen delivery to the patient, and can provide both respiratory and cardiac support. As venous blood is drained and the oxygenated return is directed back into the arterial system, recirculation does not occur. VA ECMO results in higher oxygen saturations in patients with respiratory failure than VV support, as more native cardiac output is drained from the venous system and bypasses the damaged pulmonary circuit. VA cannulation induces afterload on the left ventricle, and can quickly result in a weak ventricle failing to be able to open the aortic valve. This "cardiac-stun" effect can result in left atrial hypertension and pulmonary edema or hemorrhage. This manifests clinically by poor perfusion, and loss of pulsatility in the arterial waveform. Afterload may be reduced with medications or low-dose inotropes may improve myocardial performance to allow ejection to occur. Decompression of the left side of the heart is often accomplished in children by creating a communication (septostomy) between the left and right atrium to allow drainage by the venous cannula into the ECMO circuit. Other ways to decompress the left side of the heart include a cannula placed transseptally, a cannula placed directly into the left atrium (direct cannulation via central ECMO), or an Impella device. The Impella device (Abiomed, Inc, Danvers, MA) is a catheter-based device that has an inlet port, a motor, and an outlet port. The device can be placed femorally or axillary, and has the potential to increase hemolysis during ECLS if used at the higher settings. Currently, the Impella device is limited to older children and adults because of the length of the motor to the catheter tip. Generally speaking, the distance from the aortic valve to the apex of the ventricle needs to be approximately 7 cm to safely place this device.

Flow rate estimates for patients will help determine cannula and tubing sizes. Although estimating cardiac output can be done based on routine formulas, general guidelines suggest 100 mL/kg for neonates and 80 mL/kg for pediatric patients. Those with conditions of high oxygen consumption, such as septic shock, or dual circulations, such as Blalock-Taussig shunts, for hypoplastic left heart syndrome may require doubling of estimated flow. Some patients with high oxygen delivery requirements may benefit from transitioning from peripheral to central cannulation to obtain the greatest ECMO flow.

Common diagnoses and outcomes for neonatal and pediatric patients are shown in **Tables 3** and **4**. In neonates, congenital diaphragmatic hernia remains a lesion with the worst prognosis. Despite many efforts to improve outcome, survival averages 50%. For pediatric patients, comorbidities are now common in many patients, including cancer. Although outcome in these patients is lower than in those without such conditions, survival rates of 30% to 60% still can be attained. Most cardiac patients are postoperative from repair of congenital heart disease, but myocarditis, cardiomyopathies, arrhythmias, poisonings, and other diseases are increasingly a part of the cardiac ECMO population. One thing that remains clear in postoperative patients is that lack of myocardial recovery within 72 hours is a poor prognostic sign. Cardiac catheterization to identify residual defects that can be ameliorated should be undertaken early in the course of patients who are not recovering quickly. By one week, discussion of suitability for listing for heart transplantation should occur. One exception to the quick recovery scenario is myocarditis, whereby patients may be supported for weeks before cardiac recovery occurs. Some centers will transition patients from ECMO to ventricular assist devices (VADs) for long-term bridging to transplantation or recovery, but the cost involved

Table 3
Pediatric respiratory runs by diagnosis: ELSO registry report, January 2017

Diagnosis	Total Runs	Average Run Time	Longest Run Time	Survived	% Survived
Viral pneumonia	1756	317	2968	1150	65
Bacterial pneumonia	786	285	1411	469	59
Pneumocystis pneumonia	36	369	1144	19	52
Aspiration pneumonia	334	241	2437	227	67
ARDS, postop/trauma	199	244	935	125	62
ARDS, not postop/trauma	605	307	3086	331	54
Acute respiratory failure, non-ARDS	1437	269	7503	802	55
Other	2827	229	2699	1460	51

Abbreviations: ARDS, acute respiratory distress syndrome; ELSO, Extracorporeal Life Support Organization.

in use of VADs must be weighed against the benefit, especially in centers with low volumes. Studies have shown that heart transplant recipients who received ECMO before transplantation have lower survival compared with those bridged directly from VADs.

One increasing population for ECMO support is in patients with refractory cardiac arrest (extracorporeal cardiopulmonary resuscitation [ECPR]). Although outcome in these patients averages 40% survival to hospital discharge in children, given that survival would be zero in those not responding to conventional CPR, perhaps this is encouraging. Shorter duration of CPR has been associated with better outcome in some reports and made no difference in others. Likely, quality of CPR before ECMO is most important rather than time. Recent data showing no benefit from hypothermia in either out-of-hospital or in-hospital arrest may change this aspect of postarrest care. In any case, prevention of arrest and need for ECPR should be the goal; case reviews often identify warning signs that were missed in the pre-ECPR period.

Table 4
Cardiac runs by diagnosis: ELSO registry report, January 2017

Diagnosis	Total Runs		Survived		% Survived	
	Neonate	Pediatric, >28 d and <18 y	Neonate	Pediatric, >28 d and <18 y	Neonate	Pediatric, >28 d and <18 y
Congenital defect	5908	5371	2356	2545	39	47
Cardiac arrest	93	281	30	120	32	42
Cardiogenic shock	114	309	48	165	42	53
Cardiomyopathy	143	816	86	490	60	60
Myocarditis	88	443	44	315	50	71
Other	714	1922	336	1021	47	53

Abbreviation: ELSO, Extracorporeal Life Support Organization.

Patient Care

The goal of ECMO is to provide adequate gas exchange and oxygen delivery to allow time for the underlying disease process to resolve. Following surrogates for oxygen delivery, such as hemodynamics, acidosis, lactate, venous saturations, urine output, perfusion, and organ function parameters should be mandatory aspects of care. Setting goals for adjustment to pump flow to maintain adequate oxygen delivery should be set and discussed with the team daily. Weaning should occur as soon as adequate gas exchange at nontoxic ventilator levels and cardiac performance with minimal vasoactive requirement is achieved.

Hypertension is one common problem, especially in VA ECMO.[7,8] A decrease in cardiac filling pressures due to decompression of the atria by the ECMO circuit can reflexively cause tachycardia and hypertension. Some may treat this with antihypertensives, but care must be taken because this can exacerbate the hypertension/tachycardia, as using vasodilators can decrease preload and subsequently further decrease the filling pressures.

In the setting of septic shock, higher ECMO flows (150–200 mL/kg per minute) may be required to meet the demands of high-output cardiac failure. Careful consideration must be given before cannulation to determine if these flows can be achieved peripherally. If these flows cannot be achieved via peripheral cannulation, then central cannulation should be considered.[9]

INDICATIONS AND CONTRAINDICATIONS

The indications for initiating extracorporeal support on a critically ill child is an ever-expanding field. General guidelines from the ELSO Web site are outlined in **Table 5**. Patient populations who were previously considered absolute contraindications are now being considered relative contraindications; however, if the patient has a nonsurvivable disease process with no ability to bridge to something else (transplant), then most would consider that a contraindication. There are no specific respiratory indications for ECMO, but it is best if initiated earlier (<14 days and preferably <7 days of high

Table 5
Extracorporeal membrane oxygenation indications and contraindications

Indications	Relative Contraindications	Contraindications
• PaO_2-FiO_2 ratio: <60–80 • Oxygen Index >40 • Mean airway pressure >20–25 on conventional ventilation or >30 on HFOV • Evidence of iatrogenic barotrauma • Acute unremitting hypercapnic or hypoxic respiratory failure • Air leak syndrome • Mediastinal masses • Pulmonary embolism • Cardiac failure • Cardiac arrest	• Duration of pre-ECLS mechanical ventilation >14 d • Recent neurosurgical procedures or intracranial hemorrhage (<7 d) • Preexisting chronic illness with poor long-term prognosis • Allogeneic bone marrow transplant recipients • Solid organ tumors	• Lethal chromosomal abnormalities (Trisomy 13 or 18) • Severe neurologic compromise (intracranial hemorrhage with mass effect) • Incurable malignancy

Abbreviations: ECLS, extracorporeal life support; HFOV, high frequency oscillatory ventilation; PaO_2-FiO_2, partial pressure of oxygen dissolved in blood–fractional inspired oxygen.

ventilator support).[10,11] Although the oxygen index and partial pressure of oxygen dissolved in blood (PaO_2)-FiO_2 ratio has been used by some as criteria for initiation of ECMO, this has never been validated as a definitive indication for pediatric ECMO. Extracorporeal life support also has found a place in the algorithm for management of acute respiratory distress syndrome (ARDS), septic shock, and ECPR when traditional CPR has failed.

VENTILATOR MANAGEMENT

Ventilator management during ECMO support remains controversial. ELSO publishes broad guidelines regarding ventilation. These include minimal "rest" settings with low-rate, long inspiratory time, plateau pressure less than 25 cm H_2O, low fraction of inspired oxygen less than 0.4, and positive end-expiratory pressure (PEEP) set at an appropriate level for patient condition.[12] The paucity of literature on this subject leads many centers to develop their own individual strategies. Historically, 2 main strategies have permeated the culture: a lung open (recruitment) strategy that uses higher levels of PEEP[13–15] versus a lung rest strategy that focuses on spontaneous breathing and low PEEP.[16] One older neonatal study found shorter duration of ECMO and fewer complications in patients with PEEP levels of 12 to 14 versus 3 to 5 cm H_2O.[17]

An increasingly popular choice among ECMO centers in the era of "awake" ECMO is managing the patient extubated. This helps to minimize adverse effects of ventilator-associated lung injury and minimize sedation needs. This is also now in the ELSO guidelines.[12] In a study by Pilar Anton-Martin and colleagues,[18] patients receiving ECMO were successfully managed extubated without any adverse effects, and in cases of respiratory compromise, such as ARDS, the lungs recruited spontaneously. A recent unpublished survey (completed in 2016) of ECMO centers from around the world demonstrated that many more centers are extubating their patients. Of the centers that participated in the survey, at total of 40% reported extubating their patients, and 27% of pediatric ECMO centers reported extubating their patients. This is in contrast to a survey published in 2014 by Marhong and colleagues[19] that reported fewer than 2% of all ECMO centers were extubating patients who received ECMO.

PHARMACOLOGY

Not much is known concerning what really happens to medications after circulating through the ECMO circuit. Placing a patient on ECMO will increase the volume of distribution and can deplete plasma proteins. Thus, medications that are protein mode or have a small volume of distribution will be affected the most. Medication levels may decrease as a result of hemodilution or adherence to the ECMO circuit.

Sedation and Analgesia

The goal of sedation on ECMO should be patient comfort and safety, but at the same time minimizing the adverse effects of narcotics, benzodiazepines, and other medications; however, these practices vary widely among ECMO centers with no clear benefit of one sedative/analgesic over another. The amount of sedative as well as the actual sedative choice continues to be a moving target. Common analgesic medications given during ECMO support are fentanyl and morphine. This is partially due to the ubiquitous use in intensive care units, and because many patients placed on ECMO are already on these infusions. In general, these medications have become first-line agents at many institutions. Both of these medications are lipophilic and will be sequestered by the circuit.[20] This may necessitate a bolus during initiation of ECMO. One stated advantage of morphine over fentanyl is that morphine is believed to be less bound to the circuit than fentanyl, and some have suggested it be used for long-term sedation and analgesia in the management of patients receiving ECMO.[20] Common sedative medications are benzodiazepine infusions. Midazolam, a commonly used benzodiazepine, is also lipophilic, and can be sequestered by the circuit. Increased doses may be necessary for sedation.[21]

An increasingly popular choice for sedation is a centrally active alpha agonist, such as dexmedetomidine. Very little is known about the effects of dexmedetomidine during ECLS. One study demonstrated that dexmedetomidine is not sequestered by the oxygenator, but is, in fact, absorbed by polyvinyl chloride tubing.[22] Another sedative that has been used is propofol. This sedative had fallen out of favor due to propofol infusion syndrome and concerns for adverse oxygenator interactions.[23] With the newer iterations of oxygenators, propofol no longer has any major adverse effects on the oxygenator itself, and a recent study by Hohlfelder and colleagues[24] showed that propofol may actually extend the oxygenator life.

ANTICOAGULATION MANAGEMENT
Anticoagulation

Anticoagulation can be a great challenge for the ECMO provider. For purposes of discussion, the more commonly chosen anticoagulants are discussed as well as some of the newer ones. Heparin is the most commonly used anticoagulation medication for patients receiving ECMO. Many centers will use a bolus of heparin of 50 to 100 U/kg before cannula placement.[4] Many centers will have primed the circuit with heparin in addition to the heparin bolus. It antagonizes antithrombin III to produce its anticoagulation effect. It is excreted via the renal route, and can induce heparin-inducted thrombocytopenia (HIT) for which the medication has to be stopped. Although many tests (activated clotting time, anti-Xa level, partial thromboplastin time [PTT], thromboelastography) are being used to follow and titrate anticoagulation, none have been shown to be superior to another, but each of them may be more useful than the others based on your patient's condition. An alternative to heparin if HIT occurs is bivalirudin, which is a direct thrombin inhibitor that is gaining increasing popularity. Bivalirudin is synthetically similar to hirudin (leech saliva). Therapeutic monitoring of bivalirudin is by the direct thrombin inhibitor (DTI) assay (plasma-diluted thrombin time) or by the PTT, but the PTT is less sensitive than the DTI.

Antithrombin III

Many centers will replace antithrombin if they are having difficulty achieving anticoagulation via heparin. It is unclear what thresholds should be used to replace antithrombin or if replacing antithrombin changes the overall outcome of the pediatric patient. In fact, there is evidence to suggest that antithrombin replacement can increase thrombotic and hemorrhage complications during ECLS support.[25,26] The most common method of replacement is intermittent, but some centers have used a continuous infusion of antithrombin.[27]

FLUID OVERLOAD AND RENAL DYSFUNCTION

Fluid overload during ECLS is a common problem faced by many ECMO practitioners. In a recent multicenter report from the kidney intervention during ECMO study group, 60% of pediatric patients on ECMO had acute kidney injury (AKI).[28] This study also found that presence of AKI was associated with longer duration of ECMO and increased adjusted odds of mortality at hospital discharge.[28] **Table 6** outlines the

Table 6
Renal complications: ELSO registry report, January 2017

	% Reported		% Survived	
Diagnosis	Pediatric Respiratory	Pediatric Cardiac	Pediatric Respiratory	Pediatric Cardiac
Creatinine 1.5–3.0	8.7	10.2	35	32
Creatinine >3.0	4.1	4.1	34	33
Dialysis required	10.9	9.1	33	26
Hemofiltration	23.2	22.0	48	41
CAVHD	9.0	7.1	40	36

Abbreviation: CAVHD, continuous arteriovenous hemodialysis; ELSO, Extracorporeal Life Support Organization.

latest ELSO registry percentage of renal dysfunction, and need for dialysis for respiratory and cardiac failure. With some of the recent literature that points to an increase in mortality with fluid overload, many ECMO providers are aggressive in controlling their patient's fluid status.[29] The reasons for fluid overload stem from multiple factors: continuous infusions that make elimination by normal kidneys challenging, renal dysfunction that further complicates the kidneys' ability to keep up with the fluid input, and capillary leak from the patient's underlying condition or from the circuit that leads to third spacing and fluid overload. Three main strategies exist to help with this problem. A common first-line strategy is diuretic therapy. If urine output is inadequate, then either slow continuous ultrafiltration (SCUF) or continuous renal replacement (CRRT) may be used.

SCUF is the removal of fluid from the circuit, but renal clearance is unreliable via this method. If reliable renal replacement is needed, then CRRT becomes more advantageous. This can have the advantage of providing hemodialysis, convective clearance, or both. Such an approach is recommended by nephrologists and seems physiologically sound. The CRRT pump can be integrated into the ECMO circuit or run separately through a dialysis catheter. The disadvantage is cost and possibly increasing the risk of hemolysis and thrombocytopenia.[30,31] Some have used CRRT to help with clearance of proinflammatory cytokines, but whether this is beneficial to patients receiving ECMO remains to be seen.[32]

WEANING FROM EXTRACORPOREAL SUPPORT

Weaning from ECMO support should be a consideration from day 1 with the known complications associated with the therapy. One of the main considerations should be the reversal of the underlying disease process for which the patient was placed on ECMO. However, this may not be the case when the consideration should be if the patient can be supported as a bridge to transplantation. Weaning of VA and VV support are outlined in **Table 7**.

NUTRITION

Nutrition is very important in the management of pediatric patients receiving ECMO. In a recent study by Anton-Martin and colleagues,[33] underweight patients receiving ECMO had a higher mortality than did other patients. In their study, if the weight z score was less than −2, the inpatient hospital mortality for patients receiving

Table 7 Weaning of VA and VV support	
VA	**VV**
• Remove or clamp the LA vent • Optimize ventilation • Optimize fluid balance • Decrease ECMO flows by 10–20 mL/kg/min to 40–50 mL/kg/min • Obtain ECHO during decreased flows • Clamp trial (7–10 min at a time), "Flash" and continue clamp trail • If tolerating the clamp trial, then obtain ECHO	• Optimize ventilation • Decrease Fio$_2$ • Decrease sweep gas • Consider weaning the ECMO flows • "Cap" the oxygenator • Remember that it will take at least 20 min for the membrane lung to de-gas.

Abbreviations: ECHO, echocardiogram; ECMO, extracorporeal membrane oxygenation; ELSO, Extracorporeal Life Support Organization; Fio$_2$, fractional inspired oxygen; VA, venoarterial; VV, venovenous.

ECMO was 65.8%.[33] This necessitates optimizing nutrition for these patients, but the main problem is how to optimize nutrition.

Although total parenteral nutrition used to be a popular choice, it is often not necessary after the patient has been stabilized.[34] In the American Society for Parenteral and Enteral Nutrition clinical guidelines for neonatal ECMO, recommendations were to start nutritional support expeditiously and enteral nutrition to be initiated when the patient is clinically stable.[35] In patients who cannot tolerate gastric feeding, a postpyloric tube may be placed at the bedside under fluoroscopic guidance to ameliorate the risk of injury. As extubation and tracheostomy placement during ECMO are increasingly becoming popular, some patients may be able to tolerate oral feeds.

HEMOLYSIS AND PLASMAPHERESIS

Hemolysis can be a difficult problem to control, as there are many theories as to why it occurs in patients receiving ECMO. Another problem with hemolysis is actually defining diagnostic criteria. One might use plasma-free hemoglobin (PFH) as a marker of hemolysis. According to ELSO, a PFH greater than 50 mg/dL should be investigated.[12] The management of hemolysis includes limiting revolutions per minute,[31] minimizing negative venous pressure,[9,36] minimizing "chattering or chugging,"[31] minimizing additional circuits,[30] and possibly maintaining hemoglobin level at 13 mg/dL or less.[36] Plasmapheresis has been used in the nontransplant patient population as well as in patients receiving ECMO to reduce circulation inflammatory mediators.[4] Although some might use plasma exchange for hemolysis,[37] there remains no literature to support or refute its use in this way during ECLS. The decision to initiate plasma exchange for hemolysis in these patients should remain an individualized decision based on experience, provider knowledge, and locally based ECLS protocols.

COMPLICATIONS (EXCERPTED FROM THE PEDIATRIC AND NEONATAL PORTION OF THE INTERNATIONAL EXTRACORPOREAL LIFE SUPPORT ORGANIZATION REGISTRY AND PEDIATRIC LITERATURE)
Bleeding

Cannula site bleeding
Bleeding at the cannula site is common (18%% respiratory and 17% cardiac) (**Table 8**), and can be managed conservatively. Most bleeding can be contained

Table 8 Hematologic complications: ELSO registry report, January 2017				
	% Reported		% Survived	
Diagnosis	Pediatric Respiratory	Pediatric Cardiac	Pediatric Respiratory	Pediatric Cardiac
GI hemorrhage	4.2	2.4	30	22
Cannula site bleeding	18.2	15.6	55	48
Surgical site bleeding	12.4	28.5	47	44
Hemolysis	10.4	9.4	47	37
DIC	5.4	3.8	26	28

Abbreviations: DIC, disseminated intravascular coagulation; ELSO, Extracorporeal Life Support Organization; GI, gastrointestinal.

with pressure and reinforcing the dressing at the site. Topical coagulants also have been used with some success.

Surgical site bleeding
Bleeding at the surgical site is more common in cardiac (29%) than respiratory (12%) ECMO (see **Table 8**). Some might start an antithrombolytic infusion and decrease the heparin infusion before starting the surgery to help ameliorate the postoperative bleeding. Some have opted to stop the anticoagulation 6 hours before the procedure and the restart it 6 to 24 hours after the procedure.[38]

Gastrointestinal hemorrhage
Gastrointestinal hemorrhage (see **Table 8**) is not common (4% respiratory and 2% cardiac), but can be devastating to the patient receiving ECMO. Many times it is due to trauma from a nasogastric tube insertion or a predisposing condition (such a gastritis). A reduction in anticoagulation medication is not typically indicated, and optimizing antireflux medications may be beneficial.

Cardiac tamponade
Tamponade (2% in respiratory and 5% cardiac) may impair venous return, and cause problems with ECMO flows. If the patient has an open chest or chest tubes, a reduction in the chest tube output or a bulge in the chest patch should prompt the clinician to evaluate the patient for tamponade by either a bedside ultrasound or a formal echocardiogram.

Central nervous system complications
Cerebral hemorrhage is arguably the most feared complication of ECLS. Intracranial bleeding overall is approximately 10% (6% in respiratory and 5% cardiac) with higher rates of bleeding in neonates by the latest ELSO registry report. Many pediatric patients are cannulated in the neck (such as internal jugular and carotid), which may increase the risk of central nervous system complications. Cerebral embolism generally arises from ECMO circuit clots, which can easily pass into the aortic arch and subsequently travel to the cerebral vasculature. Seizure, either clinical or subclinical by electroencephalogram, is a well-known complication particularly in the neonatal population (**Table 9**). It remains unclear whether near infrared spectroscopy (NIRS) during ECMO can tell us whether or not the brain is suffering injury, but there do appear to be regional differences during multisite NIRS that may reflect ongoing damage.[39]

Table 9
Central nervous system complications: ELSO registry report, July 2016

Diagnosis	% Reported		% Survived	
	Pediatric Respiratory	Pediatric Cardiac	Pediatric Respiratory	Pediatric Cardiac
Brain death: clinically determined	4.4	4.3	—	—
Seizures: clinically determined	4.9	6.1	36	27
Seizures: EEG determined	1.6	2.4	37	34
CNS infarction by imaging	4.2	5.0	35	36
CNS hemorrhage by imaging	6.4	5.3	23	26

Abbreviations: CNS, central nervous system; EEG, electroencephalogram; ELSO, Extracorporeal Life Support Organization.

Infection

Perhaps one of the more difficult problems to deal with is infection (17% respiratory and 11% cardiac). Infection can occur in any central line, at the cannula insertion site, possible manufacture contamination of the cannulas or other ECMO equipment, or seeded infection from the underlying sepsis. The typical markers of infection, such as C-reactive protein and procalcitonin (PCT), are unreliable.[40] In fact, PCT levels can paradoxically be lower in ECMO-infected patients.[40]

Mechanical Complications

Premature de-cannulation

This is most likely to occur during transport of the patient to another area of the hospital (ie, to radiology for a computerized tomography scan). Transferring the patient receiving ECMO to a stretcher, to another hospital bed, or within the hospital is the most vulnerable time that this can occur. Extubated or undersedated patients may pull the cannulas out themselves. Prevention by good communication among the entire team before moving the patient, ensuring a cooperative patient, and providing adequate sedation in a noncooperative patient are effective means to help reduce this risk. Despite concerns, inadvertent de-cannulation occurs rarely if good practice is followed.

Membrane lung failure

Membrane lung failure is another problem (10% respiratory and 7% cardiac), and usually happens slowly over the course of a couple of days to weeks. A loss of both oxygenation and carbon dioxide exchange will be noted. A widening pressure gradient across the oxygenator also can be observed as clots build up within the membrane lung and increase resistance to blood flow. Water vapor buildup also can decrease efficiency and periodic "sighing" of the membrane lung by increasing the sweep gas flow can help eliminate water buildup. If failing, the membrane lung can be replaced itself, or the entire circuit changed. Often, if the membrane lung is failing, clots are also present in the entire circuit and changing the circuit may be most expeditious.

Tubing rupture

Tubing rupture occurs more frequently with the roller pumps (raceway rupture <1% respiratory and cardiac). Other causes of tubing rupture can include closing doors or a bed wheel transecting the tubing (2% respiratory and <1% cardiac). Whatever the cause of the tubing rupture, the management includes replacing the circuit.

Pump malfunction

Pump malfunction is not common (2% respiratory and cardiac). If there is a manufacturer defect, certainly the pump can stop working. A secondary pump is typically at the bedside, and can be exchanged for the defective pump. Another option is to replace the entire circuit (if desired or if using an integrated pump/oxygenator system). Most systems contain a hand-crank ability that can often allow for ECMO support when electrical failure occurs.

OUTCOMES

The overall survival to hospital discharge for pediatric respiratory ECMO is 57%. Further breakdown of survival for pediatric respiratory patients by diagnosis is listed in **Table 3**. All pediatric respiratory patients receiving ECMO should have a full neurologic examination, including some type of neurologic imaging before discharge from the hospital as well as being followed over time.[4] The overall survival to hospital discharge for pediatric cardiac ECMO is 50%. Further breakdown of survival for pediatric cardiac ECMO is listed in **Table 4**. Long-term follow-up of pediatric ECMO survivors is currently missing. In a small case series, pediatric patients with Pediatric Cerebral Performance Category (PCPC) scores show mild disabilities in 27%, moderate disability in 9%, and 9% had severe disability. In another cohort of 80 patients that included cardiac ECMO and ECPR in which plasma brain injury markers, neuroimaging, and PCPC were performed, 41% had unfavorable outcome and 31% had abnormal neuroimaging.[41]

Monitoring the ECMO program for morbidity, comparing results with national benchmark data, such as provided by the ELSO registry, and striving to become an ELSO Center of Excellence are all important goals. As technology continues to advance, ECMO and related therapies will continue to evolve. Research to reduce complications, obtain more data on both short-term and long-term outcomes and review the cost-benefit of this lifesaving but resource-heavy technology is ongoing.

REFERENCES

1. Short BL, Williams LE. ECMO specialist training manual. 3rd edition. Extracorporeal Life Support Organization; 2010. p. 1–5.
2. Bartlett RH, Roloff DW, Cornell RG, et al. Extracorporeal circulation in neonatal respiratory failure: a prospective randomized study. Pediatrics 1985;76(4): 479–87.
3. Fuhrman BP. Pediatric critical care. 5th edition. Philadelphia: Elsevier; 2017.
4. Annich G, Lynch W, MacLaren G. ECMO: extracorporeal cardiopulmonary support in critical care. 4th edition. Ann Arbor (MI): Extracorporeal Life Support; 2012.
5. Williams DC, Turi JL, Hornik CP, et al. Circuit oxygenator contributes to extracorporeal membrane oxygenation-induced hemolysis. ASAIO J 2015;61(2):190–5.
6. Dalton HJ. Venovenous extracorporeal membrane oxygenation: an underutilized technique? Pediatr Crit Care Med 2003;4(3):385–6.
7. Sell LL, Cullen ML, Lerner GR, et al. Hypertension during extracorporeal membrane oxygenation: cause, effect, and management. Surgery 1987;102(4): 724–30.
8. Makdisi G, Wang IW. Extra corporeal membrane oxygenation (ECMO) review of a lifesaving technology. J Thorac Dis 2015;7(7):E166–76.

9. Lou S, MacLaren G, Best D, et al. Hemolysis in pediatric patients receiving centrifugal-pump extracorporeal membrane oxygenation: prevalence, risk factors, and outcomes. Crit Care Med 2014;42(5):1213–20.

10. Zabrocki LA, Brogan TV, Statler KD, et al. Extracorporeal membrane oxygenation for pediatric respiratory failure: survival and predictors of mortality. Crit Care Med 2011;39(2):364–70.

11. Musick MA. Critical appraisal of Zabrocki et al: extracorporeal membrane oxygenation for pediatric respiratory failure: survival and predictors of mortality. Crit Care Med 2011; 39:364-370. Pediatr Crit Care Med 2013;14(1):85–8.

12. ELSO: Extracorporeal life support organization, Version 1.3. 2013.

13. Kacmarek RM, Villar J, Sulemanji D, et al. Open lung approach for the acute respiratory distress syndrome: a pilot, randomized controlled trial. Crit Care Med 2016;44(1):32–42.

14. Haitsma JJ, Lachmann RA, Lachmann B. Open lung in ARDS. Acta Pharmacol Sin 2003;24(12):1304–7.

15. van Kaam AH, Dik WA, Haitsma JJ, et al. Application of the open-lung concept during positive-pressure ventilation reduces pulmonary inflammation in newborn piglets. Biol Neonate 2003;83(4):273–80.

16. Camporota L, Nicoletti E, Malafronte M, et al. International survey on the management of mechanical ventilation during ECMO in adults with severe respiratory failure. Minerva Anestesiol 2015;81(11):1170–83, 1177 p following 1183.

17. Davies SW, Leonard KL, Falls RK Jr, et al. Lung protective ventilation (ARDSNet) versus airway pressure release ventilation: ventilatory management in a combined model of acute lung and brain injury. J Trauma Acute Care Surg 2015; 78(2):240–9 [discussion: 249–51].

18. Anton-Martin P, Thompson MT, Sheeran PD, et al. Extubation during pediatric extracorporeal membrane oxygenation: a single-center experience. Pediatr Crit Care Med 2014;15(9):861–9.

19. Marhong JD, Telesnicki T, Munshi L, et al. Mechanical ventilation during extracorporeal membrane oxygenation. An international survey. Ann Am Thorac Soc 2014;11(6):956–61.

20. Mousavi S, Levcovich B, Mojtahedzadeh M. A systematic review on pharmacokinetic changes in critically ill patients: role of extracorporeal membrane oxygenation. Daru 2011;19(5):312–21.

21. Chauhan S, Subin S. Extracorporeal membrane oxygenation, an anesthesiologist's perspective: physiology and principles. Part 1. Ann Card Anaesth 2011; 14(3):218–29.

22. Wagner D, Pasko D, Phillips K, et al. In vitro clearance of dexmedetomidine in extracorporeal membrane oxygenation. Perfusion 2013;28(1):40–6.

23. Ng GW, Leung AK, Sin KC, et al. Three-year experience of using venovenous extracorporeal membrane oxygenation for patients with severe respiratory failure. Hong Kong Med J 2014;20(5):407–12.

24. Hohlfelder B, Szumita PM, Lagambina S, et al. Safety of propofol for oxygenator exchange in extracorporeal membrane oxygenation. ASAIO J 2017;63(2):179–84.

25. Wong TE, Nguyen T, Shah SS, et al. Antithrombin concentrate use in pediatric extracorporeal membrane oxygenation: a multicenter cohort study. Pediatr Crit Care Med 2016;17(12):1170–8.

26. Byrnes JW, Swearingen CJ, Prodhan P, et al. Antithrombin III supplementation on extracorporeal membrane oxygenation: impact on heparin dose and circuit life. ASAIO J 2014;60(1):57–62.

27. Agati S, Ciccarello G, Salvo D, et al. Use of a novel anticoagulation strategy during ECMO in a pediatric population: single-center experience. ASAIO J 2006; 52(5):513–6.
28. Fleming GM, Sahay R, Zappitelli M, et al. The incidence of acute kidney injury and its effect on neonatal and pediatric extracorporeal membrane oxygenation outcomes: a Multicenter Report from the Kidney Intervention during Extracorporeal Membrane Oxygenation Study Group. Pediatr Crit Care Med 2016;17(12): 1157–69.
29. Lex DJ, Toth R, Czobor NR, et al. Fluid overload is associated with higher mortality and morbidity in pediatric patients undergoing cardiac surgery. Pediatr Crit Care Med 2016;17(4):307–14.
30. Betrus C, Remenapp R, Charpie J, et al. Enhanced hemolysis in pediatric patients requiring extracorporeal membrane oxygenation and continuous renal replacement therapy. Ann Thorac Cardiovasc Surg 2007;13(6):378–83.
31. Toomasian JM, Bartlett RH. Hemolysis and ECMO pumps in the 21st century. Perfusion 2011;26(1):5–6.
32. De Vriese AS, Colardyn FA, Philippe JJ, et al. Cytokine removal during continuous hemofiltration in septic patients. J Am Soc Nephrol 1999;10(4):846–53.
33. Anton-Martin P, Papacostas M, Lee E, et al. Underweight status is an independent predictor of in-hospital mortality in pediatric patients on extracorporeal membrane oxygenation. JPEN J Parenter Enteral Nutr 2016. [Epub ahead of print].
34. Ferrie S, Herkes R, Forrest P. Nutrition support during extracorporeal membrane oxygenation (ECMO) in adults: a retrospective audit of 86 patients. Intensive Care Med 2013;39(11):1989–94.
35. Jaksic T, Hull MA, Modi BP, et al, American Society for Parenteral and Enteral Nutrition (A.S.P.E.N.) Board of Directors. Clinical guidelines: nutrition support of neonates supported with extracorporeal membrane oxygenation. JPEN J Parenter Enteral Nutr 2010;34(3):247–53.
36. Jenks C, Potter D, Zia A, et al. 400: risk factors for hemolysis on ECMO: a comparison between centrifugal and roller pumps. Crit Care Med 2015;43(12 Suppl 1):101–2.
37. Hei F, Irou S, Ma J, et al. Plasma exchange during cardiopulmonary bypass in patients with severe hemolysis in cardiac surgery. ASAIO J 2009;55(1): 78–82.
38. Lamb KM, Cowan SW, Evans N, et al. Successful management of bleeding complications in patients supported with extracorporeal membrane oxygenation with primary respiratory failure. Perfusion 2013;28(2):125–31.
39. Tian F, Jenks C, Potter D, et al. Regional cerebral abnormalities measured by frequency-domain near-infrared spectroscopy in pediatric patients during extracorporeal membrane oxygenation. ASAIO J 2016. [Epub ahead of print].
40. Rungatscher A, Merlini A, De Rita F, et al. Diagnosis of infection in paediatric veno-arterial cardiac extracorporeal membrane oxygenation: role of procalcitonin and C-reactive protein. Eur J Cardiothorac Surg 2013;43(5): 1043–9.
41. Bembea MM, Rizkalla N, Freedy J, et al. Plasma biomarkers of brain injury as diagnostic tools and outcome predictors after extracorporeal membrane oxygenation. Crit Care Med 2015;43(10):2202–11.

Extracorporeal Membrane Oxygenation Management

Techniques to Liberate from Extracorporeal Membrane Oxygenation and Manage Post–Intensive Care Unit Issues

Joseph B. Zwischenberger, MD[a],*, Harrison T. Pitcher, MD[b]

KEYWORDS

- Decannulation • Weaning • Complications • Rehabilitation • Palliative

KEY POINTS

- Once extracorporeal membrane oxygenation (ECMO) has been established, attention must be directed toward optimizing recovery, minimizing complications, minimizing end-organ damage, and ultimately weaning patients from ECMO support.
- Detailed understanding of the weaning process and application of validated weaning techniques can greatly improve patient outcomes.
- Post-ECMO patients often require physical, occupational, and speech therapy in addition to assistance with nutritional issues.
- Recent studies have shown that both physical and emotional domains improved with longer follow-up after ECMO.

INTRODUCTION

Extracorporeal membrane oxygenation (ECMO) is a life-saving technique used in circumstances when patients require pulmonary and/or cardiac support for days to weeks for recovery, bridge to decision, or transplantation.[1] Over the past several decades, ECMO has evolved to provide cardiopulmonary support to patients recovering from lung failure; heart failure; trauma; acute arrest; and pretransplantation, during transplantation, or post–cardiac transplantation or post-lung transplantation in both children and adults. More recently, ECMO has been used for temporary

Disclosure: Dr J.B. Zwischenberger receives royalties from Avalon-Maquet for his licensed patent on the double lumen cannula he coinvented.
[a] Department of Surgery, University of Kentucky College of Medicine, 800 Rose Street, MN264, Lexington, KY 40536-0298, USA; [b] Thomas Jefferson University, 925 Chestnut Street, Mezzanine, Philadelphia, PA 19107, USA
* Corresponding author.
E-mail address: jzwis2@uky.edu

Crit Care Clin 33 (2017) 843–853
http://dx.doi.org/10.1016/j.ccc.2017.06.006
0749-0704/17/© 2017 Elsevier Inc. All rights reserved.
criticalcare.theclinics.com

support to allow diagnostics, recovery, or determination of eligibility or availability of a suitable donor organ. Decades of publications and educational materials have addressed the management of ECMO in different settings and populations. Little has been written regarding post-ECMO management and optimal rehabilitation of the ECMO survivor. In many ways, the post-ECMO period recapitulates the entire field of critical care.

COMPLICATIONS

As ECMO continues to evolve so does its safety profile. Nevertheless, it remains an invasive therapy with requirement for extracorporeal circulation of the patient's blood volume to remove carbon dioxide and oxygenate red blood cells before returning blood to the patient's body. Caregivers must be particularly vigilant to prevent or minimize the complications that may arise while a patient is on ECMO to lessen the burdens of post-ICU care.

WEANING FROM EXTRACORPOREAL MEMBRANE OXYGENATION

Due to the complications associated with ECMO, as discussed previously, it is best to keep patients on ECMO as little time as necessary to accomplish recovery, a bridge to destination therapy, transplant, or withdrawal. Patients can potentially be on ECMO for several days to weeks to months. As the technology of ECMO has improved and complications have decreased, the risk/benefit of longer ECMO runs has improved. Recruitment maneuvers should be performed prior to the weaning trial to optimize lung function. Also, according to Extracorporeal Life Support Organization guidelines, hepatic function should have recovered prior to any attempt to wean patients from ECMO, irrespective of the findings of cardiac assessment. Once a patient demonstrates good performance with no support from the oxygenator, the cannulas may be removed, either percutaneous (with pressure) or open (with direct vascular control or repair). Either can be done at the bedside or in the operating room with the patient sedated and monitored. In an international survey that analyzed 141 responses from 283 Extracorporeal Life Support Organization–registered ECMO centers contacted across 28 countries, 90% of the centers favored weaning patients from the ECMO circuit before weaning from the ventilator.[2]

Weaning protocols at the authors' center have been streamlined to a standardized method. The principles of weaning from ECMO no matter the etiology require the following pre-weaning parameters: clear chest radiograph, afebrile, euvolemia, and resolution/treatment options (left ventricular assist device [LVAD], total artificial heart [TAH], and transplantation) of the first problem. Failure to respect the principles results in unsuccessful outcomes.

Weaning from VV support in the setting of respiratory failure alone is somewhat subjective but involves an amalgamation of the data derived from a patient's overall pulmonary performance from current ventilator parameters, including oxygen requirements, compliance, and radiologic evidence of resolution of the initial insult. The goal of weaning should be successful conversion to conventional modes of ventilatory support without the need for ECMO support.

In the circumstances of dual system failure, such as cardiac stunning secondary to a hypoxic event, successful weaning involves encompassing a combination of both approaches. Regardless of which mode of support is weaned from, the primary mandate remains that there must be resolution of the original organ system insult to allow for ongoing physiologic stability without ECMO support or an alternative capability to take over its function. An example is transition to an LVAD from VA-ECMO in the setting of unresolved left ventricular (LV) dysfunction in the appropriate candidate.

Weaning from venovenous–extracorporeal membrane oxygenation

The methods for weaning from venovenous (VV)-ECMO differ from those for venoarterial (VA)-ECMO (**Table 1**). Based on the type of ECMO, multiple breathing tests are usually done prior to the discontinuation of ECMO to confirm that the heart and lungs are ready. For years, measures of respiratory mechanics served as a surrogate to determine a patients' ability to breathe on their own. These measures have included minute ventilation, vital capacity, maximum inspiratory force (also called negative inspiratory force), and respiratory rate.

VV-ECMO trials are performed by eliminating all countercurrent sweep gas through the oxygenator. Circuit flow does not need to be reduced, and extracorporeal blood flow remains constant so no additional heparin is required.[3] Systemic arterial oxygen saturation and pCO_2 should be monitored closely, and lung ventilation should be increased to ensure adequate CO_2 clearance as indicated by arterial and venous blood gas results. The authors observe patients for 4 hours to 24 hours with ventilation at nonharmful settings and the gas flow to the ECMO circuit at 0 L/min. If parameters remain stable, patients are ready to be removed from VV-ECMO.

Weaning from venoarterial–extracorporeal membrane oxygenation

Formal weaning studies must be performed to ascertain if a patient's heart is capable of circulatory support without VA-ECMO. VA-ECMO weaning trials require temporary clamping of both the drainage and infusion lines, while allowing the ECMO circuit to circulate through a bridge between the arterial and venous limbs. This prevents thrombosis of stagnant blood within the ECMO circuit. In addition, the arterial and venous lines should be flushed continuously with heparinized saline or intermittently with heparinized blood from the circuit. Once the native circulation can be sustained by the native heart, gas flow is reduced from 2.5 L/min by 0.5 L/min increments while assessing both hemodynamic and echocardiographic changes, and lung ventilation is increased. In general, VA-ECMO trials are shorter in duration than VV-ECMO trials because of the higher risk of thrombus formation. Once cardiac function is improved,

Table 1 Difference in methods for weaning from venovenous–extracorporeal membrane oxygenation differ from those for venoarterial–extracorporeal membrane oxygenation	
Venovenous	**Venoarterial**
• Maintain ECMO flow rate	• Heparin so activated clotting time >400 to decrease risk clotting
• Re-establish patent's full ventilation	• Decrease pump flow 1 L while ventricular function assessed by TEE
• Turn off O_2 to oxygenator	• Period of low-flow ECMO before decannulation ○ Respiratory function is a concern: turn off gas flow (only at circuit flows ≤1.5 L/min) and assess oxygenation achieved using the ventilator exclusively. Note: in this situation, the circuit flow acts as a right-to-left shunt. If adequate oxygenation and CO_2 removal can be maintained in the presence of this shunt, it is likely that respiratory failure can be managed without ECMO.
• 6-h stability, then decannulation	• If O_2 good and CO_2 managed by ventilation, consider decannulation.

ECMO removal is scheduled; however, ECMO flow should be maintained above 2.5 L/min until decannulation. An algorithmic approach to weaning from VA-ECMO is outlined in **Fig. 1**.

Venoarterial Extracorporeal Membrane Oxygenation Weaning for Cardiogenic Shock

For patients who require VA-ECMO secondary to myocardial stunning from cardiogenic shock second to acute myocardial infarction, postcardiotomy failure, right ventricular (RV) failure secondary to pulmonary embolism or cardiac dysfunction, primary graft failure after cardiac transplantation, or other etiologies compromising hemodynamic stability, the anticipation is that the cardiac function will recover within a realistic time frame to allow for weaning off ECMO or as a bridge to support devices. Myocardial recovery typically occurs in the range of 7 days to 10 days. Although a majority of cases are secondary to primary LV dysfunction, the issue of interventricular dependency and secondary RV dysfunction makes information from traditional subjective trials difficult to use with standard hemodynamic monitoring. Determination of cardiac

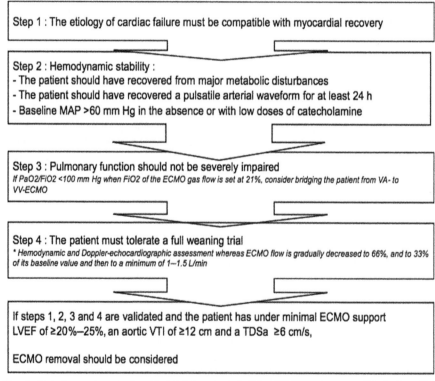

Step 1 : The etiology of cardiac failure must be compatible with myocardial recovery

Step 2 : Hemodynamic stability :
- The patient should have recovered from major metabolic disturbances
- The patient should have recovered a pulsatile arterial waveform for at least 24 h
- Baseline MAP >60 mm Hg in the absence or with low doses of catecholamine

Step 3 : Pulmonary function should not be severely impaired
If PaO2/FiO2 <100 mm Hg when FiO2 of the ECMO gas flow is set at 21%, consider bridging the patient from VA- to VV-ECMO

Step 4 : The patient must tolerate a full weaning trial
* Hemodynamic and Doppler-echocardiographic assessment whereas ECMO flow is gradually decreased to 66%, and to 33% of its baseline value and then to a minimum of 1–1.5 L/min

If steps 1, 2, 3 and 4 are validated and the patient has under minimal ECMO support LVEF of ≥20%–25%, an aortic VTI of ≥12 cm and a TDSa ≥6 cm/s,

ECMO removal should be considered

Fig. 1. Recommendations for successful weaning from VA-ECMO. CI, cardiac index; CVP, central venous pressure; LVEF, left ventricular ejection fraction; MAP, mean arterial pressure; PCWP, pulmonary capillary wedge pressure; TDS, tissue Doppler systolic velocity; VTI, velocity-time integration. (*From* Aissaoui N, Brehm C, El-Banayosy A, et al. Weaning strategy from veno-arterial extracorporeal membrane oxygenation (ECMO). In: Firsternberg MS, editor. Extracorporeal membrane oxygenation – advances in therapy. InTech Online Publishers; 2016. Available at: http://www.intechopen.com/books/extracorporeal-membrane-oxygenation-advances-in-therapy/weaning-strategy-from-veno-arterial-extracorporeal-membrane-oxygenation-ecmo.)

output using the Swan-Ganz catheter is negated by the negative pressure generated in the right atrium by the ECMO circuit; this obscures any accurate readings.[4] Real-time dynamic changes of the ventricle function during ECMO weaning would not be reflected by serial mixed venous oxygen saturation assessments, which require both the presence of a pulmonary catheter and time gaps between sampling.[5]

Failure to accurately evaluate either biventricular, or at least univentricular, recovery would carry significant potential for morbidity and mortality in any subsequent LVAD intervention. A patient assumed to have only ongoing LV dysfunction after a subjective ECMO wean failure may go on to an LVAD with a difficult and potentially fatal outcome when ongoing RV dysfunction was not recognized and the patient should have been accessed for biventricular device support or transplantation.[6] When RV failure exists in the setting of an LVAD implantation, the perioperative mortality rate increases to as high as 19% to 43%.[7] Prior to weaning the patient from ECMO, any end-organ dysfunction resulting from the pre-ECMO insult needs to be recovered to baseline.[8] Elevated lactate, significant hepatic dysfunction, and renal derangement need to be corrected. The patient needs to be afebrile and euvolemic and to demonstrate resolution of pulmonary edema on x-ray films. The fraction of inspired oxygen (FiO_2) on both the ECMO and ventilator circuits must be weaned to 50%, allowing for an acceptable upper extremity PaO_2 and saturation. The authors' institution follows an anticoagulation protocol with titration of a partial thromboplastin time (PTT) normally between 45 seconds and 55 seconds. During the weaning trial, the authors increase the PTT to 60 seconds to 70 seconds to avoid thrombotic complications while decreasing ECMO flow. The authors prefer the use of a miniaturized hemodynamic transesophageal echocardiography (hTEE) probe to access biventricular function and filling during the course of the weaning process.[9,10] The weaning process is staged to allow for progressive weaning of support while observing cardiac performance, with volume loading on reduction to half-baseline flow and finally to 1-L flow with a dobutamine drip added to demonstrate increased contractility as evidence of potential inotropic rescue if needed.

Attending ICU staff need skills to be comfortable with the use of hTEE, transthoracic echocardiogram (TTE), or transesophageal echocardiogram (TEE) and its interpretation. It is possible to follow the protocol, discussed previously, using staged bedside TTE performed by echocardiography technicians, as is the routine at many institutions. This, however, can be not only problematic from the viewpoint of availability of staff during the weaning intervals, with the weaning process taking from 4 hours to 6 hours, but also limited by the individualized body habitus of a patient, which can limit available windows for a TTE. Traditional TEE performed by a cardiologist represents an excessive commitment of resources and personnel, which is unrealistic in most hospitals. Bedside hTEE weaning has allowed the authors' center to have a positive predictive value for ventricular recovery of 100% using a standardized ECMO weaning protocol (95% CI, 73%–100%). The authors have had no major complications with the use of hTEE whereas those quoted for regular TEE are 0.2% to 0.5% per insertion. The only interval complication that has occurred has been oral-pharyngeal bleeding in a small number of patients who have required packing secondary to difficulty in passing the probe.[11–14] The weaning protocol has allowed for definitive decision making to be able to wean off ECMO, allow surgical planning to transition to an LVAD in cases of ongoing univentricular LV failure or in cases of ongoing biventricular failure transition to mechanical biventricular support or transplantation. If a patient with biventricular failure is deemed to not be a candidate for advanced mechanical support or transplantation, then appropriate preparations can be made with the family for withdrawal. The authors' weaning protocol is easily reproducible in an ICU setting and is consistently accurate. As a result, patients can be taken to an operating room for decannulation without unexpected weaning failures intraoperatively or undergo insertion of an LVAD minimizing the potential for an unpredicted need for a RV assist device or excessive inotropic in the setting of unrecognized RV dysfunction, as discussed previously. A summary of the VA weaning protocol is outlined in **Table 2**.[9]

Weaning from VV-ECMO requires the resolution of the primary issues, which may require an extended amount of time. The mantra is to be patient. The principles of weaning from VV-ECMO require the following: clear chest radiograph, afebrile, euvolemia, and resolution/treatment options (LVAD, TAH, and transplantation) of the first problem. Failure to respect the principles results in unsuccessful outcomes. The FiO_2 on both the ventilation and ECMO circuit should be weaned down to 50% or lower, with sweep less than 3 to 4 before considering weaning. The maneuvers involved in the initial weaning for VV-ECMO are (1) wean down the sweep without any increase in tidal volume, which indicates if patient lung with low volumes will remove CO_2; if successful, proceed to full weaning; (2) if step 1 is unsuccessful, wean sweep and increase tidal volumes, which should allow for adequate CO_2 removal; if successful, wean off, and, if unsuccessful, stop weaning and try another day; and (3) if step 2 is successful, wean ECMO flow down progressively while returning to standard mode of mechanical ventilation without high plateau and PEEP pressures; if successful, ECMO weaning is possible and open surgical repair is suggested for decannulation. Postdecannulation systemic inflammatory response syndrome (SIRS) has been reported to occur in approximately 60% of patients and requires attention and fever work-up. The reported observed series from the authors' group

Table 2	
venoarterial–extracorporeal membrane oxygenation weaning protocol using hemodynamic transesophageal echocardiography	
Stages of Separation	**Actions**
Prewean assessment	Prerequisite: patient is euvolemic and afebrile, chest radiograph is clear, and end-organ injury is resolved. Increase heparinization for PTT goal 60–70 s. Insert hTEE probe.
Stage 1	Baseline assessment of RV and LV functions with full ECMO flow.
Stage 2	Decrease flow from full flow to half-flow in increments of 0.5 L/min and assess LV and RV functions by hTEE over at least 0.5 h after each decrease. If distention occurs, return to full flow and abort trial.
Stage 3	Volume load (10 mL/kg)/20 min, with half-flow and assess RV and LV functions by hTEE over at least 1 h.
Stage 4	Load inotrope (dobutamine and/or milrinone), decrease flow to minimum (1–1.5/min), and assess LV and RV functions at least 1 h.
Postweaning assessment	If biventricular failure persists, consideration of end-of-life discussion should begin. If LV dysfunction persists but RV function is recovered, consider LVAD insertion. If RV dysfunction persists but LV function is recovered, consider external RV assist device. If both LV and RV functions are recovered, consider ECMO decannulation. Return to full flow and discuss timing of surgical intervention.
After weaning	Return to full flow and discuss timing of surgical intervention.

demonstrated that approximately 80% of patients had fever, approximately 70% had leukocytosis, and approximately 50% had escalation of vasopressor requirement[9] (see **Table 2**).

POST–EXTRACORPOREAL MEMBRANE OXYGENATION MANAGEMENT

After weaning from ECMO, there are still many things to be addressed. Among these are (1) potential for SIRS post-decannulation; (2) post-ECMO complications, such as deep vein thrombosis, wounds, renal failure, and stroke; (3) delirium; (4) posttraumatic stress disorder (PTSD); (5) rehabilitation; and (6) end of life.

Systemic Inflammatory Response Syndrome

SIRS is a common occurrence after ECMO. The length of time a patient's blood is exposed to the nonendothelialized surface of the cannula and extracorporeal circuit during ECMO may be responsible for the widespread activation of the innate immune system[15] and bacteremia.[16] If unchecked, inflammation and organ injury follow. Similarly, long-term ventilator support may increase the chance of ventilator associated pneumonia and subsequent development of sepsis.[5]

In a recent retrospective, single-institution study of 62 patients from Thangappan and colleagues,[17] both post-ECMO SIRS phenomenon (approximately 60%) and post-decannulation infection (approximately 60%, including infection carried over during ECMO, and approximately 35% newly developed infection after ECMO decannulation) were found common. The differentiation between SIRS and infection, however, can be difficult. In the study from Thangappan and colleagues,[17] the outcomes in patients with post-ECMO infection were poor whereas 100% of patients with SIRS only survived. Patients with suspected SIRS should be treated similarly to patients with infection with broad-spectrum antibiotics until culture results are available, and perhaps as a preventive measure antibiotics should be considered for the first 24 hours post-decannulation.

Post–Extracorporeal Membrane Oxygenation Complications

A recent meta-analysis reviewed published peer-reviewed studies related to ECMO, focusing on outcomes and complications of ECMO in adult patients; 12 studies and 1763 patients were included.[18] The most common complications associated with ECMO were found to be renal failure requiring continuous venovenous hemofiltration or short-term dialysis (occurring in 52%), bacterial pneumonia (33%), any bleeding (33%), oxygenator dysfunction requiring replacement (29%), sepsis (26%), hemolysis (18%), liver dysfunction (16%), leg ischemia (10%), venous thrombosis (10%), central nervous system complications (8%), gastrointestinal bleeding (7%), aspiration pneumonia (5%), and disseminated intravascular coagulation (5%).[18] When coming off ECMO, many patients require long-term ventilation with tracheostomy, respiratory therapy, and wound care for the various ports of entry associated with ECMO. Several studies have found, however, that both physical and emotional domains improved with longer follow-up.[19–21]

Delirium

Delirium affects mortality, length of stay, cost of care, and quality of life. As the application of ECMO has expanded, more patients are treated for weeks, even months. Such prolonged periods invite increasing opportunity for ICU delirium. Conditions that are associated with ECMO contributing to delirium include drug inducement, addiction withdrawal, sepsis, electrolyte abnormalities, nutritional deficiencies, and, in general, organ failure. Common to all ECMO is the setting for drug-induced encephalopathy. Both approaches to sedation are vulnerable. Too much sedation encourages ICU psychosis, frailty, deconditioning, deep vein thrombosis, decubitus ulcers, and other vegetative complications and increases the risk of delirium and long-term cognitive impairment.[22] Recently, enthusiasm has increased for awake and ambulatory patients on ECMO. Although many of the problems seen with over-sedation are alleviated, PTSD, discussed later, has emerged.

Several drugs are associated with anticholinergic delirium (**Table 3**).

Other common ICU medications also contribute to drug-induced delirium, including norepinephrine—α_2-agonists and opioids; serotonin—antipsychotics and antidepressants (also have anticholinergic effects); histamine—antihistamines (also have anticholinergic effects); N-methyl-D-aspartate (glutamate) antagonists—ketamine; and γ-aminobutyric acid modulators—barbiturates, benzodiazepines, hypnotics, inhalational anesthetics, and ethanol. Clearly, many opportunities exist to receive 1 or more of these drugs. Often, patients and families minimize the degree of alcohol dependency; therefore, alcohol withdrawal is also common in the ICU setting. Increasingly, recreational drug dependencies and withdrawal are seen. Sepsis is both a reason for ECMO and a complication of ECMO.

Electrolyte abnormalities are often seen during ECMO. Although total parenteral nutrition was previously associated with this problem, enteral nutrition with gastrointestinal motility and absorption abnormalities plus diuretic use often contribute to sodium imbalance. During respiratory failure, CO_2 retention has been associated with delirium, especially at levels seen with permissive hypercapnia. Organ failure can directly contribute to encephalopathy. Although outside the scope of this review, hepatic encephalopathy, uremic encephalopathy, and nutritional deficiencies (thiamine, vitamin B_6, and niacin) are all well-recognized causes of delirium that can confuse ECMO management.

Most importantly, delirium must be not only recognized but also prevented. Approaches that modify risk factors include limiting sedation with benzodiazepines, nonopioid analgesia, early mobilization, early liberation from ventilator, removal of catheters and restraints, correcting electrolytes, reducing noise and limiting exposure to artificial light at night (turn off TVs), normalizing sleep-wake cycles (preferably nonpharmacologically), encouraging social interaction, improving communication with patients, reorienting patients as needed, providing cognitive stimulation, and, finally, putting on their glasses and/or hearing aids.

Posttraumatic Stress Disorder

Current evidence from observational studies suggests that ECMO survivors have high rates of adverse mental health outcomes, including PTSD.[22–24] There are several factors that may cause a patient to develop PTSD after ECMO weaning. These include

Table 3	
Mechanism contributing to anticholinergic delirium	
Mechanism	**Examples**
Predominant muscarinic antagonists	Atropine, scopolamine, hyoscine, benztropine includes many plants
Muscarinic antagonists with other mixed effects	Antihistamines, tricyclic antidepressants, antipsychotics
Decrease acetylcholine release	Carbamazepine, opiates, cannabinoids, ethanol, Clonidine
Decrease acetylcholine synthesis	Thiamine deficiency

young age, mechanical ventilation, illness severity, drug administration, heterogeneous conditions, delirium, agitation, prolonged ICU stay, and memory of in-ICU experiences. Memory of distressing in-ICU experiences is the longest-term post-ICU PTSD risk factor.[25,26] Patients in the ICU are increasingly conscious during active treatment, and awake ECMO, in which patients are conscious, may represent a unique PTSD risk factor.[27] In the PRESERVE (Predicting the Safety and Effectiveness of Inferior Vena Cava Filters) study, data from 140 ECMO-treated acute respiratory distress syndrome patients admitted to 3 French ICUs (2008–2012) were analyzed, including health-related quality of life surveys. Health-related quality of life evaluation in 80% of the 6-month survivors revealed satisfactory mental health but persistent physical and emotional-related difficulties, with anxiety (34%), depression (25%), and PTSD (16%) symptoms reported.[25]

Although some patients only require ECMO for a few days or weeks, others have remained on ECMO and in the hospital for months. In these instances, a psychologist who interacts with patients and families is advised to help with the anxiety and stress of going through such a traumatic event.

Rehabilitation

Post-ECMO patients often require physical, occupational, and speech therapy in addition to assistance with nutritional issues. With the development of ambulatory ECMO, active rehabilitation and physical therapy can continue as patients heal or as they wait for transplantations even before weaning from ECMO. Patients who receive early rehabilitation have improved rates of return to independent functioning, decreased rates of delirium, and shorter durations of mechanical ventilation, ICU length of stay, and hospital length of stay.[25,28–31]

End-of-Life Issues

Weaning from ECMO does not always signify patient improvement or survival. Due to factors, such as age and comorbid conditions, ECMO is not always life-saving. There are times when a health care team has to discuss with patients and their families the fact that they simply cannot recover. Most hospitals that provide ECMO have a dedicated palliative care team, which becomes involved as soon as patients are put on ECMO and follows them throughout their hospitalization, in addition to providing support for patients' families.

SUMMARY

The recent success of ECMO is a consequence of both significant advances in technology of the components of the circuit as well as ECMO configuration that allows the use of ECMO in awake and ambulatory patients. The objectives are to improve the preoperative condition of the by enhancing physical strength and cardiovascular fitness and reducing the risk for post-transplant complications.

REFERENCES

1. Gattinoni L, Carlesso E, Langer T. Clinical review: extracorporeal membrane oxygenation. Crit Care 2011;15(6):243.
2. Marhong JD, Telesnicki T, Munshi L, et al. Mechanical ventilation during extracorporeal membrane oxygenation. An international survey. Ann Am Thorac Soc 2014;11(6):956–61.
3. Aissaoui N, Brehm C, El-Banayosy A, et al. Weaning strategy from veno-arterial extracorporeal membrane oxygenation (ECMO). In: Firsternberg MS,

editor. Extracorporeal membrane oxygenation – advances in therapy. InTech Online Publishers; 2016. Available at: https://www.intechopen.com/books/extracorporeal-membrane-oxygenation-advances-in-therapy/weaning-strategy-from-veno-arterial-extracorporeal-membrane-oxygenation-ecmo-.

4. Lee AJ, Cohn JH, Ranasinghe JS. Cardiac output assessed by invasive and minimally invasive techniques. Anesthesiol Res Pract 2011;2011:475151.

5. Aissaoui N, Luyt C, Leprince P, et al. Predictors of successful extracorporeal membrane oxygenation (ECMO) weaning after assistance for refractory cardiogenic shock. Intensive Care Med 2011;37:1738–45.

6. Pettinari M, Jacobs S, Rega F, et al. Are right ventricular risk scores useful? Eur J Cardiothorac Surg 2012;42:621–6.

7. Ochiai Y, McCarthy PM, Smedira NG, et al. Predictors of severe right ventricular failure. Circulation 2002;106:1198–202.

8. Wong JK, Siow VS, Hirose H, et al. End organ recovery and survival with the Quadrox D oxygenator in adults on extracorporeal membrane oxygenation. World J Cardiovasc Surg 2012;2:73–80.

9. Cavarocchi N, Pitcher H, Yang Q, et al. Weaning of extracorporeal membrane oxygenation using continuous hemodynamic transesophageal echocardiography. J Thorac Cardiovasc Surg 2013;146:1474–9.

10. Hasting HM. Transesophageal echocardiography-guided hemodynamic assessment and management. ICU Directors 2012;3:38–41.

11. Hilberath J, Oakes D, Shernan S, et al. Safety of transesophageal echocardiography. J Am Soc Echocardiogr 2010;23:1115–27.

12. Daniel W, Erbel R, Kasper W, et al. Safety of transesophageal echocardiography: a multicenter survey of 10,419 examinations. Circulation 1991;83:817–21.

13. Kallmeyer D, Collard C, Fox J, et al. The safety of intraoperative transesophageal echocardiography: a case study of 7200 cardiac patients. Anesth Analg 2001;92:1126–30.

14. Min J, Spencer K, Furlong K, et al. Clinical features of complications from transesophageal echocardiography: a single –center series of 10,000 consecutive examinations. J Am Soc Echocardiogr 2005;18:925–9.

15. Wang S, Krawiec C, Patel S, et al. Laboratory evaluation of hemolysis and systemic inflammatory response in neonatal nonpulsatile and pulsatile extracorporeal life support systems. Artif Organs 2015;39(9):774–81.

16. Haneke F, Schildhauer TA, Schlebes AD, et al. Infections and extracorporeal membrane oxygenation: incidence, therapy, and outcome. ASAIO J 2016;62(1):80–6.

17. Thangappan K, Cavarocchi NC, Baram M, et al. Systemic inflammatory response syndrome (SIRS) after extracorporeal membrane oxygenation (ECMO): incidence, risks and survivals. Heart Lung 2016;45:449–53.

18. Zangrillo A, Landoni G, Biondi-Zoccai G, et al. A meta-analysis of complications and mortality of extracorporeal membrane oxygenation. Crit Care Resusc 2013;15(3):172–8.

19. Herridge MS, Cheung AM, Tansey CM, et al. One-year outcomes in survivors of the acute respiratory distress syndrome. N Engl J Med 2003;348(8):683–93.

20. Herridge MS, Tansey CM, Matte A, et al. Functional disability 5 years after acute respiratory distress syndrome. N Engl J Med 2011;364(14):1293–304.

21. Schmidt M, Zogheib E, Roze H, et al. The PRESERVE mortality risk score and analysis of long-term outcomes after extracorporeal membrane oxygenation for severe acute respiratory distress syndrome. Intensive Care Med 2013;39(10):1704–13.

22. Takala J. Of delirium and sedation. Am J Respir Crit Care Med 2014;189(6): 622–4.
23. Brechot N, Luyt CE, Schmidt M, et al. Venoarterial extracorporeal membrane oxygenation support for refractory cardiovascular dysfunction during severe bacterial septic shock. Crit Care Med 2013;41(7):1616–26.
24. Mirabel M, Luyt CE, Leprince P, et al. Outcomes, long-term quality of life, and psychologic assessment of fulminant myocarditis patients rescued by mechanical circulatory support. Crit Care Med 2011;39(5):1029–35.
25. Risnes I, Heldal A, Wagner K, et al. Psychiatric outcome after severe cardiorespiratory failure treated with extracorporeal membrane oxygenation: a case-series. Psychosomatics 2013;54(5):418–27.
26. Jones C, Bäckman C, Capuzzo M, et al. Precipitants of post-traumatic stress disorder following intensive care: a hypothesis generating study of diversity in care. Intensive Care Med 2007;33(6):978–85.
27. Rattray JE, Johnston M, Wildsmith JA. Predictors of emotional outcomes of intensive care. Anaesthesia 2005;60(11):1085–92.
28. Tramm R, Hodgson C, Ilic D, et al. Identification and prevalence of PTSD risk factors in ECMO patients: a single centre study. Aust Crit Care 2015;28(1):31–6.
29. Schweickert WD, Pohlman MC, Pohlman AS, et al. Early physical and occupational therapy in mechanically ventilated, critically ill patients: a randomised controlled trial. Lancet 2009;373(9678):1874–82.
30. Burtin C, Clerckx B, Robbeets C, et al. Early exercise in critically ill patients enhances short-term functional recovery. Crit Care Med 2009;37(9):2499–505.
31. Morris PE, Goad A, Thompson C, et al. Early intensive care unit mobility therapy in the treatment of acute respiratory failure. Crit Care Med 2008;36(8):2238–43.

Issues in the Intensive Care Unit for Patients with Extracorporeal Membrane Oxygenation

Hitoshi Hirose, MD, PhD[a],*, Harrison T. Pitcher, MD[b],
Michael Baram, MD[c], Nicholas C. Cavarocchi, MD[b]

KEYWORDS

- Intensive care • ECMO • Circulation • Ventilator management • End-organ failure

KEY POINTS

- Extracorporeal corporeal oxygenation (ECMO) flow should be maintained to perfuse and recover the end organs.
- Ventilator management involves lung protective ventilator strategies.
- Anticoagulation during ECMO should be appropriately monitored.
- Near-infrared tissue oximetry is an important tool to assess cerebral and limb perfusion.

INTRODUCTION

Critically ill patients require very thorough physical and laboratory assessments to address medical and surgical issues. Patients on extracorporeal corporeal oxygenation (ECMO) support require an additional level of attention. Much of the focus for these patients revolves around cardiovascular support or ventilator needs. The effects of multiorgan dysfunction syndrome can ravage ECMO patients and require multiple levels of support beyond the traditional cardiovascular support. Special consideration must be given to heart–vasopressor–lung–ventilator–ECMO interactions, but that is not all. Attention must be given to patients requiring renal support to correct metabolic derangements. Hepatic support may be necessary to mitigate the effects of hepatic failure. Clinicians must understand that ECMO is a support system to allow organs

Disclosures: None for any author.
[a] Department of Cardiothoracic Surgery, Thomas Jefferson University Hospital, 1025 Walnut Street, Room 605, Philadelphia, PA 19107, USA; [b] Department of Cardiothoracic Surgery, Thomas Jefferson University Hospital, 1025 Walnut Street, Room 605, Philadelphia, PA 19107, USA; [c] Division of Pulmonary and Critical Care Medicine, Thomas Jefferson University Hospital, 834 Walnut Street, Room 650, Philadelphia, PA 19107, USA
* Corresponding author.
E-mail address: Hitoshi.Hirose@jefferson.edu

Crit Care Clin 33 (2017) 855–862
http://dx.doi.org/10.1016/j.ccc.2017.06.007
0749-0704/17/© 2017 Elsevier Inc. All rights reserved.

to recover, and patients often get worse before they get better. This article addresses select topics of intensive care unit rounds that arise on ECMO patients. The topics covered in this article should be considered in routine rounding to be sure that the patient is maximally supported once a patient is committed to ECMO support.

CARDIAC CIRCULATION

End-organ perfusion can be defined by blood flow and pressure. To maintain end-organ perfusion, the blood pressure goal of the patients on venoarterial (VA) or venovenous (VV) ECMO should be maintained at a mean arterial pressure of 65 to 70 mm Hg or higher, like other critically ill patients.[1,2] The mean arterial pressure of patients on VA ECMO should be controlled at less than 100 mm Hg owing to competition of systemic vascular resistance, left ventricular (LV) afterload and distention, and ECMO flow. Optimum ECMO flow should be determined by unloading of the ventricles, not solely based on a body surface area (BSA) times 2.2.[3] Our previous review suggested that a higher mean arterial pressure improved survival, but liberal use of vasopressors to achieve a mean arterial pressure goal is yet to be proven. Tissue perfusion is the goal of flow and pressure, with confirmation by both physical (eg, urine output) and laboratory (eg, lactate) parameters.

Cardiac function should be monitored by transthoracic echocardiography or continuous hemodynamic transesophageal echocardiography. In case of cardiac standstill, cardiac decompression needs to occur within 4 to 6 hours before worsening pulmonary edema and LV distention occur. Options for the medical management of cardiac arrest or pulseless electrical activity on ECMO should include full ECMO flow, decreased systemic resistance, correction of temperature, electrolytes, acidosis, and hypoxia, and/or inotropes. Failure of return of pulsatility will mandate the use of surgical vents to decompress the LV cavity and prevent pulmonary edema. Cardiac standstill increases the incidence of blood stasis in the ventricle, which increases the risk of the stroke.[4] All inotropes should be discontinued as soon as the VA ECMO is started, to decrease the myocardial work and allow the VA ECMO to maintain the circulation. An intraaortic balloon pump may interfere with the ECMO flow and not decrease the LV afterload, but will increase diastole filling; it is recommended to remove if the coagulation profile is reasonable.[5] The cardiologists' routine use of the Impella 2.5 to unload the LV before ECMO may be excessive and costly, with minimal benefits and significant risks of hemolysis and displacement or perforation. Swan Ganz monitoring on patients on ECMO is not necessary. The pulmonary artery and central venous pressure are not accurate and it may depend on the ECMO flow.

Maximum ECMO flow is usually determined by cannula. Each cannula has a specific flow–pressure curve. The larger cannula is able deliver a larger flow. For example, a 17-F arterial cannula is only able to provide 4 to 5 L/min, whereas a 21-F arterial cannula can provide 6 L/min without adding extreme pressure on the cannula.

Besides mechanical issue of the cannula size, low ECMO flow can occur anytime during ECMO. Low ECMO flow often results in low perfusion pressure, low end-organ perfusion, hypoxemia, hypercapnia, and worsening of shock. Thus, a low ECMO flow should be addressed immediately. The low flow is usually related patient volume status and frequently observed within 24 hours after ECMO initiation, or observed during aggressive diuresis. Before low ECMO flow, "line chattering" is often observed. Line chattering is the phenomenon that venous cannula hit against venous wall owing to negative pressure created by the ECMO circuit because of low intravascular volume status.[6] Continuous chatter may cause the ECMO to alarm or "suck down," which can be resolved quickly by dialing down the ECMO flow until there is minimal chatter; slowly increasing the ECMO flow will stabilize the flow as we infuse fluid. Volume administration is essential to resolve this issue. If low flow persists, the clinician should assess for possible sources of fluid loss, such as bleeding into the retroperitoneal cavity, gastrointestinal bleeding, third spacing into surgical wounds, or venous cannula malposition. In VA ECMO, if the venous cannula is located in the inferior vena cava with low ECMO flow, the tip of cannula needs to be advanced at least to the right atrium and preferably to the superior vena cava to maximize flow. In VV ECMO, the clinician should investigate cannula migration to either the right ventricle or the hepatic vein by radiographic and echocardiographic imaging, followed by immediate cannula reposition.[7,8] Other considerations of the low flow status, despite volume administration, are venous cannula compression abdominal distention, tension pneumothorax, pericardial tamponade, or large thrombus formation on the cannula.[9]

PULMONARY

Once a patient is initiated on ECMO, the ventilator transitions from a tool that supports oxygenation and ventilation to a tool that reduces systemic inflammation.[10] While on ECMO, the lungs still provide a small component of the gas exchange, but ventilator strategy is critical to avoid overdistention or underdistention and injury. With the reduced reliance on the lung while on ECMO (either VA or VV), the ventilator management converts to a lung-protective strategy by reducing tidal volumes to or below the 6 mL/kg of ideal body weight.[11–13] Although low tidal volume management for lung protection is standard, decreasing driving pressure (the pressure different between peak pressure [positive end-expiratory pressure]) across the lung and avoiding derecruitment, which is critical to recovery.[14] Lungs that derecruit require high pressures to overcome atelectasis, which is to overcome the natural hysteresis that occurs with hypoventilation. The resulting increased pressure and loss of surfactant can contribute to worse inflammation. Thus, the positive end-expiratory pressure needs to be adjusted based on individual peak airway pressure. Because ECMO can provide oxygen directly to the blood, the inspired fraction of oxygen (FiO_2) through the ventilator can be minimized to reduce oxygen toxicity.[15] Although there is no consensus about the exact goals or best mode of ventilation while on ECMO, traditional oxygenation targets are typically Po_2 of greater than 60 mm Hg and O_2 saturation of greater than 80% mm Hg.

Consolidations of the lungs are commonly seen in patients on ECMO for acute respiratory distress syndrome. Patients with posterior consolidations most likely have a benefit from prone positioning.[16] There are no randomized studies on proning ECMO patients; however, there are many centers that prone patient on ECMO.[17] Experience with proning patients using a Rotaprone bed (KCI, San Antonio, TX) to control the proning time have been undertaken successfully, with strict attention to securing the ECMO circuit, endotracheal tube, and other intravenous lines. Proning can be considered as an adjuvant to ECMO low tidal ventilation. If thick or high amount of secretion is present, bronchoscopy often be necessary for pulmonary toileting.

The ECMO oxygenator needs to be checked daily for clots or white fiber threading. Poor oxygenation may occur owing to exhaustion of the oxygenator. The oxygenator failure can be confirmed by preoxygenator and postoxygenator blood gas analysis. If there is less than 150 mm Hg difference between the preoxygenator and postoxygenator Pao_2 with an Fio_2 of 100% via ECMO, oxygenator change should be considered.[18]

METABOLIC

Liver and renal functions should be improved after placement of ECMO, as end-organ perfusion is improved by ECMO.[19] Deterioration of renal and liver function may be a sign of ECMO malfunction or preexisting renal or liver disease.[20] Continuous renal replacement therapy is recommended as a separate circuit from ECMO to avoid air emboli. Persistent acidemia could be owing to lack of perfusion to any organ, tissue necrosis, or distal limb ischemia. Oxygenator exhaustion may present as massive hemolysis.[21] The differential between hematuria (treatment could be holding anticoagulation), disseminated intravascular coagulopathies, and hemolysis (treatment could be increase the anticoagulation) needs urgent workup, because treatment is important.

GASTROINTESTINAL

Enteral feeding is the preferred route of nutrition.[22] When ECMO patients require paralytics in addition to sedation, a postpyloric feeding tube is recommended.[23] In case of the patients requiring prone position, bridling the feeding tube may be necessary. Sudden abdominal distension or an increase in lactate may be early signs of ischemic bowel, which may result in poor prognostic signs.[24] Oral–pharyngeal bleeding is common in ECMO patients owing to the multiple instrumentations such as transesophageal echocardiography or feeding tube placement. An appropriate consultation with an ENT specialist and packing may be required; surgical intervention is necessary in approximately 20% of the cases due to a laceration.[25]

The overall incidence of acute liver failure during ECMO is approximately 15%, with cases of acute liver failure progressing into multiorgan failure and death.[26] In our institution, we advocated utilization of liver dialysis (a molecular adsorbent recirculating system) if patients developed rising bilirubin (>10 mg/dL) or an acute increase in liver enzymes (>1000 IU/L) despite appropriate ECMO flow and blood pressure.[27]

VASCULAR

Vascular complications are common and indications of poor outcomes in patients on VA ECMO.[28] To avoid vascular complications, distal perfusion catheter placement is recommended in all cases in VA ECMO and cannulation should be done under fluoroscopy and ultrasound guidance.[29] The distal femoral perfusion catheter enters the femoral artery distal to the arterial ECMO cannula and provides oxygenated blood to the distal limb. It is needed owing to the restriction of blood down the femoral artery due to the presence of arterial cannula. Patency confirmation of the distal perfusion port is important and may require an angiogram. The distal perfusion catheter may become clotted, dislodged, or malpositioned, resulting in ischemic limb complications. Routine pulse checks using Doppler ultrasound should be performed. To ensure distal limb perfusion, lower extrimity tissue oximetry should be routine in the care of patients on VA ECMO support.[3,18]

HEMATOLOGY

Anticoagulation should be initiated on postoperative day 1 with heparin with a goal partial thromboplastin time (PTT) of 45 to 55 seconds.[30] There are various assays used to monitor anticoagulation including anti-factor X, activated clotting time, and PTT; PTT is the most cost effective at the bedside. In our institution, 5000 to 7500 U of the heparin are administered at the time of cannulation and the heparin drip begins on post-ECMO day 1. Our anticoagulation goal is PTT 45 to 55 seconds in VA and VV ECMO.[31] If the patient develops bleeding complications, anticoagulation can be safely held with full ECMO flow.[19] If active bleeding is observed, the heparin drip can be held 6 hours for minor bleeding, and could be held for additional 24 hours in case of major bleed, such as ongoing retroperitoneal, gastrointestinal, or endotracheal bleeding. Surgical or interventional corrections of the bleeding site should be considered.[31] On VV ECMO, anticoagulation can be held for a prolonged time period, because the risk of stroke is not related to the circuit. On VA ECMO, a prolonged period of no anticoagulation may place on the patient risk of thromboembolism. If thromboembolism were expected owing to low ECMO flow, cardiac standstill, or a history of pulmonary emboli, the anticoagulation goal should be increased to a PTT of 50 to 65 seconds. The ECMO circuit must be monitored continuously for thrombi and fibrin formation. The circuit exhaustion is usually observed by the poor oxygenation from the oxygenator rather than low ECMO flow, as described. If the oxygenator needs to be changed, no additional bolus of heparin is necessary.

The hemoglobin should be kept at greater than 8 to 9 g/dL to optimize oxygen delivery. A decrease in hemoglobin may occur at the time of initiation of ECMO owing to hemodilution from the circuit. The ECMO circuit volume could be minimum 400 mL depending on the length of the tubing and circuit design. A persistent decrease in hemoglobin shortly after cannulation could indicate major vascular injury and a prompt imaging study may be necessary.

Platelet consumption by the pump can be observed, and is tolerated with no bleeding and a platelet count of greater than 50,000 (B/L). If heparin-induced thrombocytopenia is suspected, platelet factor 4 (PF4) assay and serotonin release assay (SRA) should be performed and a hematology consult may be necessary before switching to alternate anticoagulants, which are costly.[32]

INFECTION

After perioperative period, antibiotics should not be necessary unless other identified infection are present. ECMO patients are at risk for infections acquired in the intensive care unit, including line access infections, Foley catheter infections, and ventilator-associated pneumonia. The systemic inflammatory response can also occur with fever and leukocytosis on ECMO,[33] but all fevers require workup. The question of starting empiric antibiotics (after all cultures are done) is further assessed by using a procalcitonin assay. Our previous study showed that the procalcitonin level was highly correlated with the presence of infection.[34] We believe procalcitonin-driven antibiotic therapy could be cost effective; culture results take a maximum of 5 days, whereas procalcitonin results are available on same day of the sampling. A procalcitonin level of greater than 5 mg/dL should prompt a workup for infection and empirical treatment with broad-spectrum antibiotics.[34] Daily assessment of the cannulation site, routine aseptic dressing change of the cannulation site, and minimizing movement of the cannula should be routine in the care of the patient on ECMO support.

Postdecannulation systemic inflammatory response syndrome has been reported to occur in approximately 60% of patients and requires attention and fever workup. The reported observed series from our group demonstrated that approximately 80% of patients had fever, approximately 70% had leukocytosis, and approximately 50% had escalation of vasopressor requirement.[36] Patients with culture-proven infection have lower survival rates.[36]

NEUROLOGIC

Neurologic injury is a devastating complication of ECMO and a frequent cause of death on ECMO support.[35] Thromboembolism can originate from the aorta, cannulation site, or ECMO circuit. Anticoagulation may contribute to the risk of the intracranial bleeding. Hypoxia or low cerebral perfusion either during or before ECMO may result in anoxic brain injury.

During ECMO support, the majority of patients are deeply sedated making complete neurologic examinations difficult, despite daily sedation vacation. Cerebral oximetry using near-infrared spectroscopy is an important tool to identify the low cerebral perfusion and may be useful for early detection of neurologic injury.[3] The regional oxygen saturation (rOS_2) should be monitored during ECMO. Decreases in rOS_2 values to less than 40 or a decrease of rOS_2 values of more than 20% from baseline could be significant; this depends on the device being used and it normal readings. A bilateral decrease of rOS_2 could reflect a systemic event such as low perfusion pressure and/or hypoxia, which should be immediately treated by increasing the perfusion pressure and flow, as well as the oxygen by ECMO or ventilator, and checking the hemoglobin concentration.[3] A unilateral decrease in the rOS_2 or persistent bilateral decrease in the rOS_2 despite these treatments most likely indicates a cerebral ischemic event.[3] Prompt computed tomography scanning is necessary to rule out neurologic injury.

INPATIENT TRANSPORT

During ECMO support, transporting the patient through the hospital may be necessary. The patient may go to the operating room, CT scan, to interventional radiology, or catheterization laboratory for various reasons. These transports should be done with standard monitoring by a qualified team including nursing, a perfusionist, and a respiratory therapist. Although our ECMO program does not require the routine presence of a perfusionist at the bedside, the perfusionist should accompany all ECMO transports in case of a mechanical problem.[37] Pump stoppage is rare but can be occur during transport. If ECMO stops running, hand cranking must initiate without delay. While 1 person continues hand cranking for the ECMO, a perfusionist can either reset the ECMO machine or bring a new circuit.

FAMILY INVOLVEMENT

Explaining to family members the procedure, risks, and benefits of ECMO support is difficult for many physicians, particularly regarding how to emphasize that ECMO is a support device for recovery, treatment, or withdrawal. Giving family members hope but realistic goals is difficult in these urgent situations. Nursing and other staff taking care of the patient should also explain the ECMO circuit and ensure the necessity of the ECMO in laymen language. We should emphasize the ECMO is not standard therapy, and the patient's circulation and oxygenation and CO_2 removal depend on the circuit. It is important to update the family daily and to review the options for outcome, such as full or partial recovery, the need for a durable cardiac support device for bridge to decision, futility, or long-term need for transplantation. Social work, care management, religious workers, and palliative care all have a role in ensuring the well-being of the family.

REFERENCES

1. Leone M, Asfar P, Radermacher P, et al. Optimizing mean arterial pressure in septic shock: a critical reappraisal of the literature. Crit Care 2015;19:101.
2. Magder SA. The highs and lows of blood pressure: toward meaningful clinical targets in patients with shock. Crit Care Med 2014;42:1241–51.

3. Wong JK, Smith TN, Pitcher HT, et al. Cerebral and lower limb near-infrared spectroscopy in adults on extracorporeal membrane oxygenation. Artif Organs 2012; 36:659–67.

4. Unai S, Nguyen M, Tanaka D, et al. Clinical significance of spontaneous echo contrast on extracorporeal membrane oxygenation. Ann Thorac Surg 2017;103: 773–8.

5. Park TK, Yang JH, Choi SH, et al. Clinical impact of intra-aortic balloon pump during extracorporeal life support in patients with acute myocardial infarction complicated by cardiogenic shock. BMC Anesthesiol 2014;14:27.

6. Sidebotham D. Troubleshooting adult ECMO. J Extra Corpor Technol 2011;43: 27–32.

7. Chimot L, Marqué S, Gros A, et al. Avalon bicaval dual-lumen cannula for venovenous extracorporeal membrane oxygenation: survey of cannula use in France. ASAIO J 2013;59:157–61.

8. Rubino A, Vuylsteke A, Jenkins DP, et al. Direct complications of the Avalon bicaval dual-lumen cannula in respiratory extracorporeal membrane oxygenation (ECMO): single-center experience. Int J Artif Organs 2014;37:741–7.

9. Allen S, Holena D, McCunn M, et al. A review of the fundamental principles and evidence base in the use of extracorporeal membrane oxygenation (ECMO) in critically ill adult patients. J Intensive Care Med 2011;26:13–26.

10. Pipeling MR, Fan E. Therapies for refractory hypoxemia in acute respiratory distress syndrome. JAMA 2010;304:2521–7.

11. Acute Respiratory Distress Syndrome Network, Brower RG, Matthay MA, Morris A, et al. Ventilation with lower tidal volumes as compared with traditional tidal volumes for acute lung injury and the acute respiratory distress syndrome. N Engl J Med 2000;342:1301–8.

12. Thompson BT, Bernard GR. ARDS Network (NHLBI) studies: successes and challenges in ARDS clinical research. Crit Care Clin 2011;27:459–68.

13. Lehle K, Philipp A, Hiller KA, et al. Efficiency of gas transfer in venovenous extracorporeal membrane oxygenation: analysis of 317 cases with four different ECMO systems. Intensive Care Med 2014;40:1870–7.

14. Amato MB, Meade MO, Meade MO, et al. Driving pressure and survival in the acute respiratory distress syndrome. N Engl J Med 2015;372:747–55.

15. Crapo JD. Morphologic changes in pulmonary oxygen toxicity. Annu Rev Physiol 1986;48:721–31.

16. Azimzadeh N, Baram M, Cavarocchi NC, et al. Prone position: does it help with acute respiratory distress syndrome (ARDS) requiring extracorporeal membrane oxygenation (ECMO)? Open J Resp Dis 2017;7:18–24.

17. Kimmoun A, Roche S, Bridey C, et al. Prolonged prone positioning under VV-ECMO is safe and improves oxygenation and respiratory compliance. Ann Intensive Care 2015;5:35.

18. Panigada M, L'Acqua C, Passamonti SM, et al. Comparison between clinical indicators of transmembrane oxygenator thrombosis and multidetector computed tomographic analysis. J Crit Care 2015;30:441.e7-13.

19. Wong JK, Siow VS, Hirose H, et al. End organ recovery and survival with the QuadroxD oxygenator in adults on extracorporeal membrane oxygenation. Word J Cardiovasc Surg 2012;2:73–80.

20. Brodie D, Bacchetta M. Extracorporeal membrane oxygenation for ARDS in adults. N Engl J Med 2011;365:1905–14.

21. Williams DC, Turi JL, Hornik CP, et al. Circuit oxygenator contributes to extracorporeal membrane oxygenation-induced hemolysis. ASAIO J 2015;61:190–5.

22. Miessau J, Fotiou E, Cavarocchi NC, et al. Early nutritional support of patients on extracorporeal membrane oxygenation. Nutr Thera Metab 2013;31:186–91.

23. Zhang Z, Xu X, Ding J, et al. Comparison of post pyloric tube feeding and gastric tube feeding in intensive care unit patients: a meta-analysis. Nutr Clin Pract 2013; 28:371–80.

24. Schreiber J, Nierhaus A, Vettorazzi E, et al. Rescue bedside laparotomy in the intensive care unit in patients too unstable for transport to the operating room. Crit Care 2014;18:R123.

25. Harrison M, Baker A, Roy S, et al. Management of upper aerodigestive tract bleeding on extracorporeal membrane oxygenation. Mech Circulatory Support 2013;4:20333.

26. Combes A, Leprince P, Luyt CE, et al. Outcomes and long-term quality-of-life of patients supported by extracorporeal membrane oxygenation for refractory cardiogenic shock. Crit Care Med 2008;36:1404–11.

27. Sparks B, Cavarocchi NC, Hirose H. Extracorporeal membrane oxygenation with multiple-organ failure: can molecular adsorbent recirculating system therapy improve survival? J Heart Lung Transplant 2017;36:71–6.

28. Abrams D, Combes A, Brodie D. Extracorporeal membrane oxygenation in cardiopulmonary disease in adults. J Am Coll Cardiol 2014;63:2769–78.

29. Lamb K, Hirose H, Cavarocchi NC. Preparation and technical considerations for percutaneous cannulation for veno-arterial extracorporeal membrane oxygenation. J Card Surg 2013;28:190–2.

30. Lamb K, Cowan SW, Evans N, et al. Successful management of bleeding complications in patients supported with extracorporeal membrane oxygenation with primary respiratory failure. Perfusion 2013;28:125–31.

31. Pitcher HT, Harrison MA, Shaw C, et al. Management considerations of massive hemoptysis while on extracorporeal membrane oxygenation. Perfusion 2016;31: 653–8.

32. Natt B, Hypes C, Basken R, et al. Suspected heparin-induced thrombocytopenia in patients receiving extracorporeal membrane oxygenation. J Extra Corpor Technol 2017;49:54–8.

33. He C, Yang S, Yu W, et al. Effect of continuous renal replacement therapy on intestinal mucosal barrier function during extracorporeal membrane oxygenation in a porcine model. J Cardiothorac Surg 2014;23(9):72.

34. Tanaka D, Pitcher HT, Cavarocchi NC, et al. Can Procalcitonin differentiate infection from systemic inflammatory reaction in patients on extracorporeal membrane oxygenation? J Heart Lung Transplant 2014;33:1186–8.

35. Extracorporeal Life Support Organization (ELSO). Extracorporeal Life Support (ECLS) registry report international summary. 2010. Available at: https://www.elso.org/Portals/0/Files/Reports/2017/International%20Summary%20January%202017.pdf.

36. Thangappan K, Cavarocchi NC, Baram M, et al. Systemic inflammatory response syndrome (SIRS) after extracorporeal membrane oxygenation (ECMO): incidence, risks and survivals. Heart Lung 2016;45:449–53.

37. Cavarocchi NC, Wallace S, Hong EY, et al. A cost-reducing extracorporeal membrane oxygenation (ECMO) program model: a single institution experience. Perfusion 2015;30:148–53.

Staffing, Equipment, Monitoring Considerations for Extracorporeal Membrane Oxygenation

David C. Fitzgerald, MPH, CCP[a],*, Edward M. Darling, MS, CCP[b],
Monika F. Cardona, BSN, RN[c]

KEYWORDS

- Extracorporeal membrane oxygenation • Monitoring • Educational models

KEY POINTS

- Training for extracorporeal clinicians should consist of a structured and evidenced-based educational format that incorporates both didactic and applied simulation components.
- Technological advancements in current pump, oxygenator, and cannula design have not only expanded the indications of extracorporeal support, but have also been associated with an improved delivery of care.
- Continuous clinical monitoring that measures the quality and safety parameters of extracorporeal support has demonstrated significant benefits in optimizing patient care and outcome.

INTRODUCTION

Despite several early reports of the successful use of extracorporeal membrane oxygenation (ECMO) in the 1970s,[1,2] adult ECMO failed to establish itself as a conventional therapy for cardiopulmonary resuscitation. Unable to demonstrate a significant clinical benefit in randomized controlled trials, the widespread interest for adult ECMO was nonexistent for nearly 30 years while its emergence in both neonatal and pediatric applications continued.[3,4] Within the last decade, this complex, life-sustaining treatment modality has experienced exponential growth in the United States,[5] with the

The authors report no financial conflicts of interest or funding sources for this article.
[a] Division of Cardiovascular Perfusion, MUSC College of Health Professions, Medical University of South Carolina, 151B Rutledge Avenue MSC962, Charleston, SC 29425, USA; [b] Department of Cardiovascular Perfusion, SUNY Upstate Medical University, 750 East Adams Street, Syracuse, NY 13210, USA; [c] Medical University of South Carolina, 165 Ashley Avenue, CH 846, Charleston, SC 29425, USA
* Corresponding author.
E-mail address: fitzgerd@musc.edu

Crit Care Clin 33 (2017) 863–881
http://dx.doi.org/10.1016/j.ccc.2017.06.008
0749-0704/17/© 2017 Elsevier Inc. All rights reserved.

observation of similar trends occurring in adult intensive care settings across the world.[6] Not only have international, critical care teams been able to increase the use of adult ECMO but also the duration of support has been safely and significantly prolonged, maximizing any potential and realized recovery for the native heart and lungs.[7]

Although the reasons for the recent growth in adult ECMO are multifactorial, much of the success may be attributed to the development of well-trained staff and the technological innovations in equipment and monitoring devices used during extracorporeal support. In this article, the authors discuss general educational formats for the ECMO bedside provider, staffing support models, and devices designed to best meet the needs of the patient while simultaneously ensuring the proper delivery of ECMO-related care.

Educational Models for Extracorporeal Membrane Oxygenation Specialists

Historically within the world of ECMO, training models for new employees have been heavily concentrated in didactical frameworks with competency assessment through written examinations and practical application stations to facilitate demonstration of required skills. As a professional multidisciplinary organization of ECMO, the Extracorporeal Life Support Organization (ELSO) recommends a didactic training course ranging from 24 to 36 hours.[7] Specifically, ELSO guidelines recommend these didactic hours be broken down as follows: 6 to 8 hours for disease inclusion and pathophysiology, 6 to 8 hours of ECMO physiology, 4 to 8 hours for review of extracorporeal life support (ECLS) equipment/basic procedures, 4 to 8 hours of emergency management training, and a minimum of 12 hours of bedside skill review.[7] This standard educational model facilitates a very concentrated indoctrination of core ECMO principles, with minimal time allotment granted toward practical application apart from the actual patient care environment.

Although this traditional education model has proven to be successful for many programs, research has demonstrated that this specific method of instruction can become static, whereas a more "hands-on" approach is far more sustainable for the end learner.[6] The direct utilization of technology in high-fidelity simulation training fosters an educational model that is both challenging and invigorating for the learner. With the incorporation of high-fidelity simulation into ECMO education, a training model can be created that is demonstrative of an environment that is both extremely realistic and directly elicits responsiveness from participants for scenarios that are introduced.[7] The result is a valuable, true-to-life educational opportunity that can be directly translatable to performance within the actual patient care setting.[8]

The provision of an in situ setting in which ECMO clinicians can have practical application sessions is an invaluable asset to any training model.[9] The emergence of commercial hydraulic extracorporeal simulators, such as the Califia (Biomed Simulation Inc, San Diego, CA, USA) and the Eigenflow (Curtis Life Research LLC, Indianapolis, IN, USA), facilitates specific manipulations that will produce variable patient-simulated responses. Because these simulators are compatible with all types of ECMO circuits, the fidelity of the learning environment is enhanced by managing the same components that clinicians are accustomed to using in the clinical setting. The development of a training model inclusive of a realistic practice environment for clinicians enhances learning through multiple factors, such as the provision of immediate performance feedback and repetitive skill practice by the identified learner.[7] Through the purposeful placement of learners into an artificial, patient care environment, the process of simulation acts to immerse the learner and therefore is able to overcome the training deficits surrounding practical application within traditional, didactically focused training models.

ELSO now recommends the incorporation of a simulation component into any training course specific to ECMO. Simulation scenarios should be written that are relevant and applicable for the end user in the extracorporeal environment. A comprehensive offering of simulation competency assessments may include, but not be limited to, the following:

- *Low-volume and high-risk clinical duties that carry a significant risk of harm.* Examples may include ECMO pump failure, air entrainment in the circuit, and emergency support through hand-cranking.
- *Problem-prone activities that are infrequently performed and may be identified as consistent problems in performance.* Examples may include oxygenator change-out proficiency testing, intrahospital transport, and transition of care reporting.
- *Mandates for credentialing and validation to satisfy regulatory requirements.* Examples would include point-of-care device proficiency testing, blood product administration, and fire safety drills.
- *New changes in job duties, protocols, or devices.* Examples may include the orientation to new pumps, revisions to disposable circuits, or changes to clinical care policies.

In addition, simulation can be expanded beyond the scope of individual competency as a direct means to evaluate team dynamics and collaborative performance. The multidisciplinary nature of ECMO would seemingly benefit from simulation exercises aimed to improve teamwork, communication, and intraprofessional collaboration. Intense simulated emergency management in this context is of the utmost importance in the prevention of adverse outcomes in this unique and complex care delivery model.

The supplies necessary to perform simulation exercises may be obtained from expired disposable products and nonsterile materials no longer suitable for use in the patient care environment. Guidelines for the duration and frequency of simulation assessments should be documented to ensure all key stakeholders are informed and meet all departmental expectations that are in place. Competency of the ECMO Specialist can be continually assessed because knowledge application occurs in response to the predetermined testing scenarios. These crucial components must be carried out carefully to ensure the simulation education model is successful at all levels of engagement.

The observed benefits of simulation notwithstanding, there are several perceived barriers that should be addressed to optimize a high-fidelity learning environment.[10] Employers must embrace a culture that supports simulation activities outside of direct patient care schedules. This increased level of support would include capital costs for maintaining simulation equipment, staffing costs for attending and proctoring simulation, infrastructure costs for physical space and audio-video equipment, and intangible costs for developing curricula and trainers.[10]

An ECMO Program must give careful consideration to the initial training for the registered nurse and respiratory therapist desiring to enter the program to become an ECMO Specialist. This initial training should be formally structured and be accomplished through an educational format that is inclusive of both didactic and simulation components. This mixed model approach fosters the needs of the adult learner as foundational knowledge. The practical application occurs gradually throughout the learning process, further solidifying the new information acquired. Competency should be assessed not only at the conclusion of the primary training, but additionally in an ongoing manner at fixed intervals of employment. ELSO recommends an annual assessment of both cognitive and applied knowledge as part of clinical competency proficiency for both new and experienced beside ECMO care providers.[7]

Staffing models for extracorporeal membrane oxygenation patients

Within the complex and diverse community of ECMO, staffing models continue to evolve and adapt as a result of educational and technology advancements. To ensure the best possible outcome for any patient requiring this high-risk, complex modality, the collaboration of a multidisciplinary team should remain at the forefront of any structured care system.[11] Therefore, consideration in relation to models of care for this unique patient population should be ongoing and tailored to the needs of the individual ECMO center.

The primary care model used by many ECMO centers across the world is defined as a 2:1 care provider:patient ratio that is maintained throughout the entire course of ECMO.[7] This particular model uses a registered nurse with a strong critical care background and understanding of ECMO working in a synergistic, tandem capacity with the ECMO Specialist. The ECMO Specialist team may comprise ECMO trained critical care registered nurses and/or respiratory therapists, or perfusionists that have graduated from an accredited school of perfusion technology. Role delineation must occur if the bedside registered nurse does not have formal ECLS training, requiring the nurse to only perform the normal care associated with a critically ill patient in the intensive care setting. The ECMO Specialist will then hold the primary function of maintaining ECMO support encompassing circuitry, equipment, continuous assessment, and providing additional bedside assistance and expertise as needed.[7] Although this model has been proven safe and effective in many institutions, it can often be resource intensive and financially straining for adult-specific ECMO programs.[12] In these circumstances, alternative care delivery models may be considered in the provision of ECMO support.

An alternative delivery model to carefully be contemplated and considered is the single caregiver model.[7] This model is defined as an individual intensive care unit (ICU) nurse not only providing the direct nursing duties for the patient but also assuming the additional responsibilities associated with safely maintaining the ECMO system. This identified nurse must acquire additional training specific to the provision of ECMO, inclusive of circuitry, equipment, and emergency management.[7] If selected as the model of care, it is recommended to slowly transition to a 1:1 structure after initiation using a 1:1.5 ideation.[12] Proposed transition strategy should facilitate a safer transition of care during the period of time immediately after cannulation. In addition, it is strongly recommended that the clinicians assuming the role within the 1:1 structure have advanced skills surrounding the assembly, maintenance, and emergency management of the ECMO equipment used within the center.[12]

Limitations associated with the single caregiver model should be thoroughly examined before its formal institution at any ECMO center. Although proven to be extremely effective in high-volume ECMO centers because of the strain placed on staffing resources, this model can be detrimental in lower-volume centers. ECMO Specialists within these lower-volume centers may experience a significant time lapse between ECMO shift exposures. Decreased clinical exposure can limit a clinician's ability to optimally perform in expected capacities because of infrequency of cases. Robust educational programs can be implemented as direct supplements for the lack of patient contact by these clinicians; however, such programs should be strongly founded upon frequent and repetitive simulation testing.[11] Furthermore, this proposed model may not be suitable in certain disease processes, such as multisystem organ failure and acute respiratory distress syndrome, because of the complexity of care required for these patients. In these instances, centers may opt to temporarily supplement with 1:1 staffing for patients requiring higher levels of acuity. These changes in staffing models would permit patient needs to dictate the most optimum structure from which to deliver care.[11]

The ECMO rounding model has been successfully reported in busy adult cardiac surgery programs that provide high volumes of ECMO support.[13] In this model, the perfusionist serves as the ECMO Specialist, but in a more supportive and trouble-shooting role. The perfusionist rounds on each ECMO patient every 2 to 4 hours and is available on campus for emergency calls, troubleshooting, or expert consultation. By supplementing with telemetry-based electronic remote monitoring, this model permits the specialist to leave the bedside and interact with the circuit when necessary. For higher-volume ECMO centers, this model may serve as the acceptable medium between the aforementioned models, because specialists are not required to stay at the bedside for every pump, but are quickly available in acute, emergency events. The limiting factor for this model is the number of staff perfusionists available for continuous in-house ECMO support.

EXTRACORPOREAL MEMBRANE OXYGENATION EQUIPMENT

The substantial increase in the use of ECMO seen in the last decade has been facilitated by several advancements in the technology. These technological advancements include pump and pump consoles, low-resistance, long-term oxygenators, and improved cannulas. This continual evolution in ECMO circuitry has been well documented.[14–16]

The contemporary ECMO circuit, in its most basic form, consists of the following: (1) the disposable components (cannula, tubing, centrifugal pump, and polymethylpentene [PMP] oxygenator); and (2) the hardware components (a pump console that drives the pump motor and provides monitoring of various circuit technical parameters, blender/flowmeter to deliver gas though the oxygenator, and a water-bath heater to maintain normothermia).

This section describes the current technologies available in relation to pumps, oxygenators, and cannulas.

Extracorporeal Membrane Oxygenation Centrifugal Pumps and Pump Consoles

Choosing an ECMO system involves consideration of several factors: desired safety features, ease/speed of setup, cost, and the provision of direct beside ECMO support (perfusionist, ECMO specialist, bedside nurse).[17] Currently, in the United States, there are 3 primary centrifugal consoles available for ECMO usage, each associated with a specific disposable centrifugal pump head: Maquet RotaFlow (ICU package), Maquet CardioHelp, and Thoratec CentriMag. Each console is appropriate for both veno-arterial (VA) and veno-venous (VV) ECMO modes and has comparable hemolysis rates over the duration of use.[18]

Maquet RotaFlow

The RotaFlow centrifugal pump system (Maquet Getinge Group, Wayne, NJ) provides a stand-alone option for ECMO applications. The system with its companion disposable centrifugal pump is shown in **Fig. 1**. The RotaFlow disposable centrifugal pump primes with 32 mL and uses a sapphire bearing to reduce friction and heat generation. Advantages of this system include significantly lower cost compared with others, integrated flow probe and bubble detector, flow and revolutions per minute (RPM)

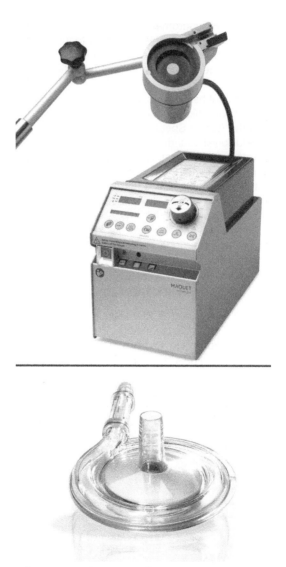

Fig. 1. Maquet rotaflow pump. (*Courtesy of* Maquet Getinge Group, Wayne, NJ; with permission.)

alarms, battery backup, and a hand crank for manual operation. One notable disadvantage is that the option is not inclusive of the ability to monitor circuit safety parameters if the ICU package is chosen to be used apart from the Heart-Lung Machine base console. These limitations in safety monitoring would include servoregulation of positive- and negative-pressure transducers, pump stoppage from air entrainment into the arterial limb of the circuit, and audible alarms for circuit temperature monitoring. Another potential disadvantage is the need to apply contact paste on the surface of the flow probe apparatus that is molded into the centrifugal pump polyvinyl chloride housing. Subsequent applications of contact paste may be necessary for prolonged support, which would require temporary interruption of patient support.

Thoratec CentriMag

The CentriMag blood pump (Thoratec Corporation, Pleasanton, CA) is approved as a modality for an right ventricular assist device (RVAD) for periods of support up to 30 days and for cardiopulmonary support up to 6 hours. The first report of the Centri-Mag being used in ECMO was by Saeed and colleagues[19] in 2007. The system with its companion disposable centrifugal pump is shown in **Fig. 2**. The centrifugal pump is unique in that its magnetically levitated impeller eliminates the need for a point contact bearing to minimize blood-related complications such as hemolysis.[20] Other advantages of this system include integrated ECMO circuit pressure monitoring capabilities, flow and pressure alarms, a pediatric-sized centrifugal pump offering ("Pedimag") that can deliver pump flows up to 1.5 L per minute, and a compact transport module weighing only 6.6 kg. A significant disadvantage is the higher cost of the pump when compared with other available centrifugal technologies in extracorporeal support. However, the difference in cost may be justified for low-volume ECMO programs, because its reported use as a short-term mechanical circulatory support (MCS) pump may be beneficial in limiting the need for maintaining numerous pump technologies.

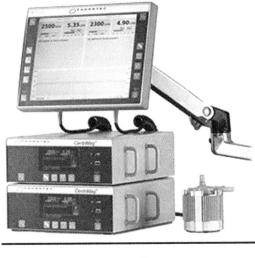

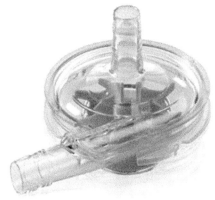

Fig. 2. CentriMag pump. (*Courtesy of* the Thoratec Corporation, Pleasanton, CA; with permission.)

The lack of a hand crank also leaves the clinician without a manual method of maintaining pump flow. As such, a console failure would potentially require prolonged interruption in support because the centrifugal pump would need to be transferred to another backup console and drive motor.

Maquet CardioHelp

Self-marketed as a portable heart-lung support system, the CardioHelp (Maquet Getinge Group, Wayne, NJ) is rapidly finding a niche in ECMO applications. The small portability of this platform along with integration of circuit pressure sensors, circuit blood temperatures, integrated measurements of the venous oxygen saturation, hematocrit, and hemoglobin makes this console a unique stand-alone platform when compared with other technologies. Also unique is the disposable component, which integrates the oxygenator heat exchanger unit into the centrifugal pump. The system with its companion disposable centrifugal pump is shown in **Fig. 3**. The advantages of this system are its portability and the comprehensive integration of circuit pressure

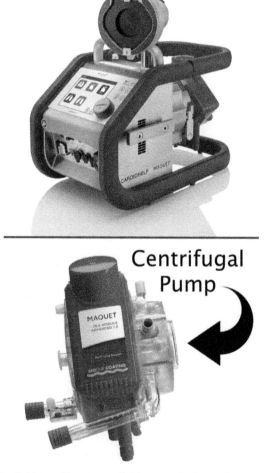

Fig. 3. Maquet CardioHelp. (*Courtesy of* Maquet Getinge Group, Wayne, NJ; with permission.)

sensors, temperature, and inline venous blood monitoring at the module. The small footprint and lightweight design is suited for interhospital transport inclusive of both road and air ambulance. The pump oxygenator base unit can be placed in an additional hand-crank unit for manual operation in the event of console failure. The console software also features an automatic priming mode that facilitates rapid deployment of emergent ECMO support. One of the perceived limitations in using the CardioHelp system are the higher hardware and disposable costs, as compared to other centrifugal pump technologies. These cost differences may be of greater significance when oxygenator change-outs are required, due to gas failure or thrombus formation. The integrated design of the centrifugal pump and oxygenator requires a complete interruption in support to accommodate a full-circuit change-out, versus an isolated oxygenator replacement.

Extracorporeal Membrane Oxygenation Oxygenators

polymethylpentene (PMP) membrane fibers are now the most common gas exchange material used in oxygenators for long-term ECMO procedures. These PMP fiber oxygenators provide adequate gas exchange and low resistance to flow and resist plasma leakage over longer periods of blood exposure.[21,22] The use of PMP fibers has resulted in fewer oxygenator change-outs as compared with previous technology found in the hollow fiber polypropylene units. In addition, the lower surface area and resistance to flow require a lower level of anticoagulation than the larger silicone-fiber membranes. To maintain normothermia, these oxygenators are also constructed with an integrated polyethylene heat exchanger that is attached to a water bath–based heater unit. Commercially, several PMP oxygenators are available in models appropriately sized from neonates to large adults. Examples are shown in **Fig. 4**. Considerations for oxygenator use include priming volume, surface area, and anticipated blood flow requirements. Oxygenators are tested and "flow rated" for the maximum blood and gas flows at which the oxygenator can receive blood at standard venous inlet condition and oxygenate it to an arterial saturation of 95%.[23] **Table 1** compares these specifications of PMP oxygenator models. Both heparin-based and nonheparin surface-modified coatings are available to limit thrombogenesis and inflammatory response during support.

Extracorporeal Membrane Oxygenation Cannula

Adequate arterial and venous cannulation is one of the most important factors in achieving *effective* ECMO therapy. Cannulas provide the critical connection between the ECMO circuit tubing and the patient's vasculature. In this regard, cannula size and position are important factors. On the venous side, a poorly positioned or an

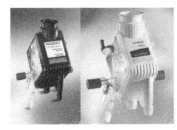
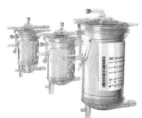
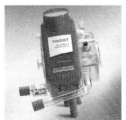

Maquet
Quadrox iD   Quadrox D

Medos
hilite 800, 2400, 7000 LT

Maquet
CardioHelp

Fig. 4. PMP oxygenators. (*Courtesy of* Xenios AG, Heilbronn, Germany; with permission.)

Table 1			
Polymethylpentene oxygenator model specifications			
PMP Oxygenator	Flow Rating (LPM)	Surface Area (m²)	Prime Volume (mL)
Maquet Quadrox D	1–7	1.8	250
Maquet Quadrox iD	0.2–1.5	0.38	38
Medos hilite 0800LT	Up to 0.8	0.32	55
Medos hilite 2400LT	Up to 2.4	0.65	95
Medos hilite 7000LT	1–7	1.9	320

Abbreviation: LPM, liters per minute.

undersized cannula can impair preload to the pump, limiting the ability to reach needed pump blood flow rates. On the arterial side, a poorly positioned or an undersized cannula can increase afterload and resistance to the pump, which also can limit pump blood flow rates. Strategies such as "triple cannulation" (VV-V, VA-V, VV-A) are ways to optimize ECMO therapy by placing an additional cannula to improve venous drainage or arterial inflow conditions.[24] Cannulas are flow rated, and the size of the cannula must be selected based on patient size and anticipated flow requirements.[25]

Dual-Lumen Venovenous Cannula

For primarily respiratory support, VV ECMO using a single dual-lumen venovenous cannula (DLVV) cannula has increased dramatically during the last decade with comparable outcomes as using conventional peripheral venous cannulation.[26] This technique is attractive because it involves a single cannulation site via the internal jugular vein for simultaneous venous drainage and reinfusion of oxygenated blood. Commercially available DLVV catheters include the Maquet Avalon Elite (Maquet Getinge Group, Wayne, NJ) and the OriGen PEBAX cannulas (Origen Biomedical, Austin, TX). Both manufacturers offer a variety of sizes to provide flow ranges appropriate for neonates to adult application (**Fig. 5**). DLVV catheters are commonly inserted via fluoroscopy and echocardiography guidance to ensure proper placement. Malposition of the cannula not only may result in increased blood recirculation in the ECMO circuit but also has been reported to cause right ventricular rupture and tamponade.[27] DLVV cannulas confer significant benefits for patients that may be candidates for ambulatory ECMO. By avoiding the use of conventional mechanical ventilation, critically ill patients that

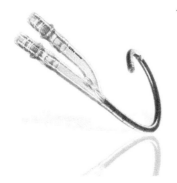
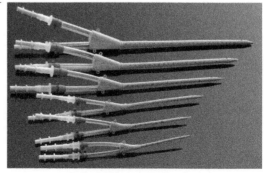

Maquet Avalon Elite   OriGen PEBAX

Fig. 5. Dual-lumen VV cannula. (*Courtesy of* Maquet Getinge Group, Wayne, NJ, and Origen Biomedical, Austin, TX; with permission.)

are awaiting lung transplantation are not required to receive excessive sedation. Ambulatory ECMO provides the opportunity for them to participate in bedside conditioning and rehabilitation as a modality to improve posttransplant outcomes.[28]

Femoral/Peripheral Cannulas

Often the VA and VV ECMO mode is accomplished percutaneously using the Seldinger technique: for VA-ECMO via femoral vein (advanced to the right atrium [RA]) and femoral artery, and for VV-ECMO via femoral vein (advanced to the inferior vena cava) and internal jugular vein (advanced to the RA). Catheter insertion kits typically include a long flexible guidewire, a scalpel, an 18-gauge insertion needle, multiple vessel dilators, and a small syringe. VA ECMO via femoral cannulation can be quickly accomplished by an experienced physician in a multitude of hospital settings. In general, cardiothoracic surgeons and cardiologists may have the most experience with catheter insertion. However, emergency department attending physicians and critical care intensivists may also be capable of initiating support. When combined with the portable design of today's ECMO pump, this seemingly infallible approach makes the initiation of adult ECMO possible across an entire hospital campus.

There are several limitations to femoral ECMO cannulation. First, obstruction of the femoral vessels from the cannulas may produce distal limb ischemia. Evaluation of distal limb flow via Doppler assessment of the pedal artery and capillary refill should be routinely performed for the entire duration of support. How regional oximetry monitoring can be used as an adjunct to diagnosing early limb ischemia is described in later discussion. Physicians may proactively insert a distal limb catheter to provide arterial blood flow beyond the femoral cannulation site. Distal limb perfusion can be achieved with an arterial catheter side-arm flowing into a small single-lumen catheter or introducer sheath advanced in the distal femoral artery.

Another limitation of peripheral cannulation may be the inability to decompress the left side of the heart during support. Distention of the left ventricle may increase pulmonary congestion and depress respiratory function. Steps in limiting LV distension may include the use of inotropic support, direct insertion of a catheter for active LV venting, transatrial balloon septostomy, or an early transition to an implantable LVAD device.

Last, the retrograde flow in the aorta from the femoral cannula may compete with the native ejection of the heart. Inadequate mixing of desaturated blood from the ventricle and fully oxygenated blood from the ECMO pump in the aorta may result in poorly saturated blood perfusing the coronary arteries and aortic arch vessels.

Neonatal VA-ECMO cannulation is typically performed via the internal jugular vein (advanced to the RA) and internal carotid artery (advanced to the aortic arch). Cannulas suitable for this application can be seen in **Fig. 6**. These cannulas are wire reinforced to prevent kinking and commonly include an introducer set with dilators to facilitate insertion. Unlike adult peripheral cannulation of the femoral vessels, the carotid artery and/or jugular vein are often ligated following ECMO decannulation.

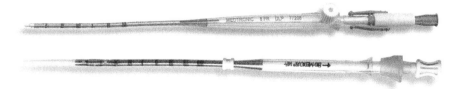

Fig. 6. Neonatal arterial and venous catheters. (Copyright (©) 2017 Medtronic. All rights reserved. Used with permission of Medtronic.)

Central Cannulation

Direct central cannulation of the aorta and right atria can be achieved through a medial sternotomy and is a suitable option for patients who fail to wean from cardiopulmonary bypass. In this scenario, cannulas are preexisting in the surgical setting and can be used through the direct connection to the ECMO circuit and console. This option may also be preferable for adult patients that do not have sufficient femoral access. The disadvantage to central cannulation for patients not requiring cardio-pulmonary bypass (CPB) is that need to perform a median sternotomy on patients that may experience functional recovery. Longer central cannulas may be able to tunnel through the skin for pump attachment, thereby allowing for chest closure after surgery. However, the patient's sternum would still require a procedural reopening if and when a conversion from ECMO is warranted.

MONITORING DEVICES FOR EXTRACORPOREAL MEMBRANE OXYGENATION SUPPORT

Continual monitoring and applicable safety devices are essential during ECMO support to not only ensure proper equipment and circuit function but also help establish an adequate level of oxygen delivery is provided to the patient's tissues.[29,30] When combined with standard ICU monitoring, these devices alert the clinicians when abnormal or unsafe conditions occur during support. Several monitoring devices can be interfaced with the ECMO console to servoregulate pump flow when the integrity of the circuit has been compromised. Furthermore, newer generation electronic medical records can record continuous output data and implement it into real-time progress report trending, quality assurance, and continuous quality improvement initiatives of the program. The following devices have conferred significant benefits in the management of safe ECMO support.

Ultrasonic Flow Probes

Continuous direct measurement of blood flow to the patient can be obtained through the utilization of an ultrasonic flow meter applied to the outflow tubing to the patient. Flow probes are commonly incorporated into the engineering design of the centrifugal head console. Although roller-head devices calculate the blood flow based on tubing diameter and pump RPM, they do not account for intracircuit shunts that direct flow away from the patient. As such, external flow probes positioned distal to all circuit shunts provide an accurate reflection of delivered extracorporeal pump flow.[31]

Extracorporeal Membrane Oxygenation Circuit Pressure Monitoring

Disposable pressure transducers may be incorporated at 3 locations of the ECMO circuit. ELSO recommends pressure monitoring of the venous drainage line, preoxygenator, and postoxygenator ports of the system.[29] Excessive negative pressure on the venous drainage catheter may traumatize the surrounding tissue of the heart and vascular endothelium as well as cause an outpouring of gaseous emboli in venous blood from tubing cavitation. Continuous negative pressure monitoring may be helpful in the assessment of intravascular volume status and proper venous catheter positioning. Positive pressure monitoring can identify high line resistance and servoregulate the pump speed to avoid circuit rupture. Oxygenator transmembrane pressure monitoring assists with the determination of the origin of high pressure. If present, it can then be directly associated with a flow obstruction in the oxygenator blood path. Elevated transmembrane pressures may signify an accumulation of fluid, thrombus, or lipids that compromise oxygenator performance.[30,32]

Oxygen Analyzers, Inline Blood Gas Monitoring, and Temperature Monitoring

External oxygen analyzers measure the percentage of fractionated oxygen gas delivered from the gas blender to the inlet port of the membrane oxygenator. Although their values should correlate closely with the fractionated inspired oxygen (FiO_2) settings on the blender, a variance between the 2 would indicate a gas source malfunction. Such a discrepancy may signify a failure of gas flow from the wall source, or a disruption of flow downstream from the blender.

Continuous inline blood-gas monitoring provides clinicians with an accurate assessment of oxygen saturation and gas exchange in real time at the point of care. Arterial and venous saturation measurements determine the delivered oxygen content and oxygen consumption from the patient. Initial calibration of these probes can be performed with laboratory blood-gas sampling from the venous and arterial output ports of the circuit. Subsequent laboratory sampling can ensure device accuracy and correlate saturation readings with oxygen partial pressure values. The CDI Blood Parameter Monitoring System 500 (Terumo Cardiovascular Systems, Ann Arbor, MI, USA) (**Fig. 7**) uses optical fluorescence to measure blood saturation, pH, Pco_2, Po_2,

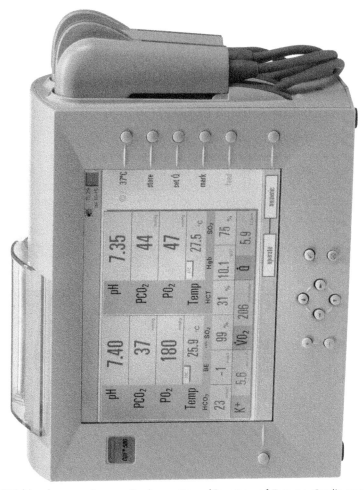

Fig. 7. CDI blood parameter monitoring system. (*Courtesy of* Terumo Cardiocascular Systems, Ann Arbor, MI; with permission.)

hematocrit, and potassium values during cardiopulmonary bypass support. Arterial and venous line sensors may be adapted into the ECLS circuit blood path to provide continuous blood parameter readings during support.[33,34] An arterial-to-venous line shunt must be incorporated into the circuit in order to use the arterial sensor probe. The M4 System (Spectrum Medical, Fort Mill, SC), depicted in **Fig. 8**, provides continuous noninvasive diagnostic measurements of oxygen saturation, hematocrit, flow and emboli detection, and ventilation diagnostics. Unlike other blood-gas technologies, none of the device sensors come in direct contact with the blood pathway. The avoidance of extra circuit connectors may reduce the risks of circuit thrombus formation and hemolysis. Overall, continuous blood-gas management during extracorporeal support has been associated with minimized parameter variation and improved blood-gas management.[35]

Temperature can be continuously monitored during support and can be measured from the patient, pump, and blood-warming device sites. Patient temperature is typically maintained at near-normothermic temperatures; however, patient temperature may be adjusted for cerebral hypoxic events, unintentional cooling and shivering, and the avoidance of hyperthermia from systemic fever.[29] Circuit temperature can be easily monitored at the blood outlet port of the membrane oxygenator. Nussmeier and colleagues[36,37] concluded that arterial blood outlet temperature serves as the closest surrogate for cerebral temperature measurement during cardiopulmonary bypass support. Despite this close association, Newland and colleagues[38] demonstrated that arterial blood temperature accuracy is not consistent across all types of membrane oxygenator manufacturers. This variation in temperature probe design may underestimate the true cerebral temperature in excess of 0.5°C.

Near-Infrared Spectroscopy

The use of cerebral and lower limb near-infrared spectroscopy (NIRS) has been reported to detect ischemic cerebral and peripheral events during ECLS support.[39–41] Patients on VA ECMO often do not produce a pulsatile blood pressure, rendering the standard pulse oximeter probes inaccurate. Unlike pulse-gate algorithms, regional

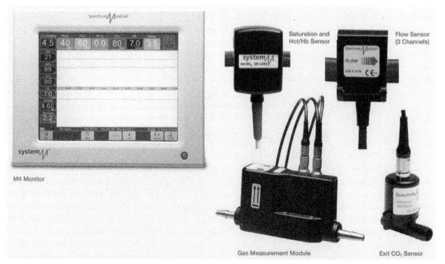

Fig. 8. M4 system. CO_2, carbon dioxide; Hb, hemoglobin; Hct, hematocrit. (*Courtesy of* Spectrum Medical, Fort Mill, SC; with permission.)

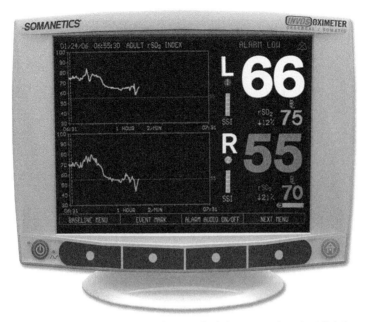

Fig. 9. INVOS cerebral/somatic oximeter. (Copyright (©) 2017 Medtronic. All rights reserved. Used with permission of Medtronic.)

oximetry technology detects the light absorption at capillary level tissue beds possessing laminar flow patterns. This modified design yields a higher venous saturation and reports a regional balance between arterial and venous tissue saturation values (**Fig. 9**). Transcutaneous adhesive sensor pads provide a noninvasive and real-time method of trending the adequacy of cerebral perfusion (**Fig. 10**). Cerebral saturation monitoring may not only prove beneficial in evaluating the global status of perfusion adequacy but also help reduce the risk of cerebral hypoxia that may be associated with peripheral VA cannulation. Arterial ECMO flow from the femoral artery catheter

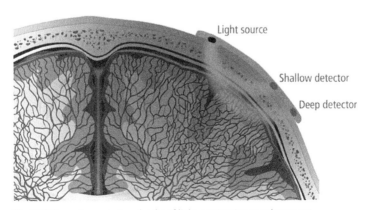

Light source

Shallow detector

Deep detector

The INVOS system uses two depths of light penetration to subtract out surface data, resulting in a regional oxygenation value for deeper tissues.

Fig. 10. INVOS cerebral/somatic oximeter sensors. (*Courtesy of* Medtronic; with permission.)

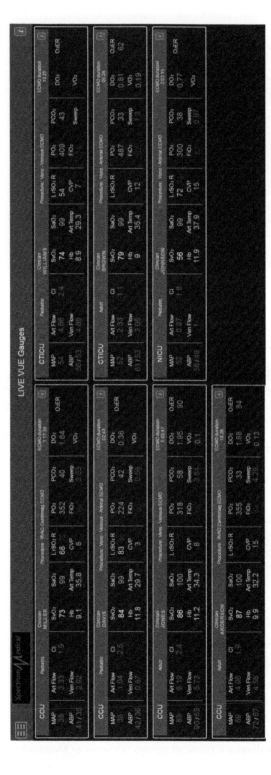

Fig. 11. Live Vue remote access tool. (*Courtesy of* Spectrum Medical; with permission.)

may compete with poorly saturated blood ejected from the native heart and lungs. This phenomenon may result in poor mixing at the level of the aortic arch and fail to achieve adequate oxygen delivery to the brain and upper extremities of the patient. Similarly, the use of NIRS has also been reported in monitoring of saturations in the lower extremities and distal limbs.[39,41] Isolated case reports and published case series describe how NIRS can be used in avoiding limb ischemia from femoral cannula obstruction. Distal limb perfusion is generally gauged using Doppler pulse sound assessment of the feet. This method may prove difficult in instances of nonlaminar flow. NIRS sensor pads placed on both legs can quantify the saturation difference in the cannulated and noncannulated legs. An early warning system for leg ischemia can provide clinicians an opportunity to insert a distal limb catheter or consider alternating their cannulation strategy. More importantly, additional diagnostic tools may prevent more severe complications such as fasciotomy and amputation.

The Future: Remote Monitoring and Telemedicine

In addition to the noted benefits of electronic data capture and reporting, newer generation technologies may pave the way to improved quality, safety, and resource utilization. Fung and colleagues[42] reported their institutional experience with the Live Vue Remote Access Tool from Spectrum Medical. Live Vue provides remote viewing of live clinical data and simultaneous viewing of multiple patients on extracorporeal support (**Fig. 11**). These critical care parameters can trigger compliance alarms that immediately alert multiple care providers of potentially adverse clinical events. By using this remote monitoring technology, Fung and colleagues[42] reported the rapid and successful deployment of staff for separate cases of acute cannula malposition and oxygenator failure. They concluded that enhanced monitoring may allow for faster staff intervention in a staff rounding model, especially in events that may not otherwise be quickly diagnosed. With the projected growth and expanding indications for ECMO support, similar telemedicine technologies may provide care teams future opportunities for remote clinical consultation and support.

REFERENCES

1. Hill JD, O'Brien TG, Murray JJ, et al. Prolonged extracorporeal oxygenation for acute post-traumatic respiratory failure (shock-lung syndrome). Use of the Bramson membrane lung. N Engl J Med 1972;286(12):629–34.
2. Bartlett RH, Gazzaniga AB, Fong SW, et al. Extracorporeal membrane oxygenator support for cardiopulmonary failure. Experience in 28 cases. J Thorac Cardiovasc Surg 1977;73(3):375–86.
3. Zapol WM, Snider MT, Hill JD, et al. Extracorporeal membrane oxygenation in severe acute respiratory failure. A randomized prospective study. JAMA 1979; 242(20):2193–6.
4. Mosier JM, Kelsey M, Raz Y, et al. Extracorporeal membrane oxygenation (ECMO) for critically ill adults in the emergency department: history, current applications, and future directions. Crit Care 2015;19:431.
5. Sauer CM, Yuh DD, Bonde P. Extracorporeal membrane oxygenation use has increased by 433% in adults in the United States from 2006 to 2011. ASAIO J 2015;61(1):31–6.
6. Lansdowne W, Machin D, Grant DJ. Development of the orpheus perfusion simulator for use in high-fidelity extracorporeal membrane oxygenation simulation. J Extra Corpor Technol 2012;44(4):250–5.

7. Ansnich G, Lynch W, MacLaren G, et al. ECMO extracorporeal cardiopulmonary support in critical care. 4th edition. Ann Arbor (MI): Extracoporeal Life Support Organization; 2012.

8. Burton K, Pendergrass T, Byczkowski T, et al. Impact of simulation-based extracorporeal membrane oxygenation training in simulation laboratory and clinical environment. Simul Healthc 2011;6(5):284–91.

9. Su L, Spaeder M, Jones M, et al. Implementation of an extracorporeal cardiopulmonary resuscitation simulation program reduces extracorporeal cardiopulmonary resuscitation times in real patients. Pediatr Crit Care Med 2014;15(9): 856–60.

10. McFetrich J. A structured literature review on the use of high fidelity patient simulators for teaching in emergency medicine. Emerg Med J 2006;23(7):509–11.

11. Park PK, Napolitano LM, Bartlett RH. Extracorporeal membrane oxygenation in adult acute respiratory distress syndrome. Crit Care Clin 2011;27(3):627–46.

12. Swol J, Belohlavek J, Haft JW, et al. Conditions and procedures for in-hospital extracorporeal life support (ECLS) in cardiopulmonary resuscitation (CPR) of adult patients. Perfusion 2016;31(3):182–8.

13. Mongero LB, Beck JR, Charette KA. Managing the extracorporeal membrane oxygenation (ECMO) circuit integrity and safety utilizing the perfusionist as the "ECMO Specialist". Perfusion 2013;28(6):552–4.

14. Palanzo D, Qiu F, Baer L, et al. Evolution of the ECLS circuitry. Artif Organs 2010; 34(11):869–73.

15. Sutton R, Salatich A, Jegier B, et al. A 2007 survey of extracorporeal life support members: personnel and equipment. J Extra Corpor Technol 2009;41:172–9.

16. Khan S, Vasavada R, Qiu F, et al. Extracorporeal life support systems: alternative vs. conventional; circuits. Perfusion 2011;26:191–8.

17. Palanzo D, Baer L, El-Banayosy A, et al. Choosing a pump for extracorporeal membrane oxygenation in the USA. Artif Organs 2014;38(1):1–4.

18. Palanzo DA, El-Banayosy A, Stephenson E, et al. Comparison of hemolysis between CentriMag and RotaFlow rotary blood pumps during extracorporeal membrane oxygenation. Artif Organs 2013 Sep;37(9):E162–6.

19. Saeed D, Kizner L, Arusoglu L, et al. Prolonged transcutaneous cardiopulmonary support for postcardiotomy cardiogenic shock. ASAIO J 2007;53:e1–3.

20. Zhang J, Gellman B, Koert A, et al. Computational and experimental evaluation of the fluid dynamics and hemocompatibility of the CentriMag blood pump. Artif Organs 2006;30(3):168–77.

21. Peek GJ, Killer HM, Reeves R, et al. Early experience with a polymethyl pentene oxygenator for adult extracorporeal life support. ASAIO J 2002;48(5):480–2.

22. Formica F, Avalli L, Martino A, et al. Extracorporeal membrane oxygenation with a poly-methylpentene oxygenator (Quadrox D). The experience of a single Italian centre in adult patients with refractory cardiogenic shock. ASAIO J 2008;54(1): 89–94.

23. FDA. Guidance for cardiopulmonary bypass oxygenators 510(k) submissions. Available at: http://www.fda.gov/OHRMS/DOCKETS/98fr/001091gl.pdf. Accessed January 12, 2017.

24. Napp JC, Kuhn C, Hoeper MM, et al. Cannulation strategies for percutaneous extracorporeal membrane oxygenation in adults. Clin Res Cardiol 2016;105: 283–96.

25. Harris WE, Darling EM, Lawson DS. ECMO equipment and devices. In: Short BL, Williams L, editors. ECMO specialist training manual. 3rd edition. Ann Arbor (MI): ELSO; 2010. p. 77–97.

26. Bittle G, Sanchez P, Pham S, et al. Veno-venous ECMO with bicaval dual-lumen catheter cannulation: a review of the ELSO registry. Crit Care Med 2015;43(12 Suppl 1):10.
27. Hirose H, Yamane K, Marhefka G, et al. Right ventricular rupture and tamponade caused by malposition of the Avalon cannula for venovenous extracorporeal membrane oxygenation. J Cardiothorac Surg 2012;7:36.
28. Lehr CJ, Zaas DW, Cheifetz IM, et al. Ambulatory extracorporeal membrane oxygenation as a bridge to lung transplantation: walking while waiting. Chest 2015;147(5):1213–8.
29. Extracorporeal Life Support Organization. General guidelines for all ECLS cases. 2013. Available at: https://www.elso.org/Portals/0/IGD/Archive/FileManager/929122ae88cusersshyerdocumentselsoguidelinesgeneralallecls version1.3.pdf.
30. Lequier L, Horton SB, McMullan DM, et al. Extracorporeal membrane oxygenation circuitry. Pediatr Crit Care Med 2013;14(5 Suppl 1):S7–12.
31. Baker RA, Bronson SL, Dickinson TA, et al. Report from AmSECT's International Consortium for evidence-based perfusion: American Society of Extracorporeal Technology standards and guidelines for perfusion practice: 2013. J Extra Corpor Technol 2013;45(3):156–66.
32. Maunz O, Penn S, Simon A. Emergency oxygenator change-out after massive fat embolism. Perfusion 2013;28(2):167–9.
33. Schreur A, Niles S, Ploessl J. Use of the CDI blood parameter monitoring system 500 for continuous blood gas measurement during extracorporeal membrane oxygenation simulation. J Extra Corpor Technol 2005;37:377–80.
34. Gelsomino S, Lorusso R, Livi U, et al. Assessment of a continuous blood gas monitoring system in animals during circulatory stress. BMC Anesthesiol 2011;11:1.
35. Ottens J, Tuble SC, Sanderson AJ, et al. Improving cardiopulmonary bypass: does continuous blood gas monitoring have a role to play? J Extra Corpor Technol 2010;42(3):191–8.
36. Nussmeier NA, Cheng W, Marino M, et al. Temperature during cardiopulmonary bypass: the discrepancies between monitored sites. Anesth Analg 2006;103:1373–9.
37. Nussmeier NA. Management of temperature during and after cardiac surgery. Tex Heart Inst J 2005;32:472–6.
38. Newland RF, Sanderson AJ, Baker RA. Accuracy of temperature measurement in the cardiopulmonary bypass circuit. J Extra Corpor Technol 2005;37:32–7.
39. Wong JK, Smith TN, Pitcher HT, et al. Cerebral and lower limb near-infrared spectroscopy in adults on extracorporeal membrane oxygenation. Artif Organs 2012;36(8):659–67.
40. Ostadal P, Kruger A, Vondrakova D, et al. Noninvasive assessment of hemodynamic variables using near-infrared spectroscopy in patients experiencing cardiogenic shock and individuals undergoing venoarterial extracorporeal membrane oxygenation. J Crit Care 2014;29(4):690.e11-5.
41. Steffen RJ, Sale S, Anandamurthy B, et al. Using near-infrared spectroscopy to monitor lower extremities in patients on venoarterial extracorporeal membrane oxygenation. Ann Thorac Surg 2014;98(5):1853–4.
42. Fung K, Beck JR, Lopez HC 2nd, et al. Case report: remote monitoring using spectrum medical Live Vue allows improved response time and improved quality of care for patients on cardiopulmonary support. Perfusion 2013;28(6):561–4.

Transport While on Extracorporeal Membrane Oxygenation Support

Kyle C. Niziolek, MD, EMT-P[a],*, Thomas J. Preston, BS, CCP, FPP[b],
Erik C. Osborn, MD[c,d]

KEYWORDS

- Extracorporeal life support (ECLS) • Extracorporeal membrane oxygenation (ECMO)
- Critical care transport • Pre-hospital • Medical evacuation

KEY POINTS

- The use of extracorporeal membrane oxygenation (ECMO) for severe acute respiratory failure has been increasing steadily.
- Evidence suggests that ECMO performed at higher volume centers is associated with improved mortality and regionalization of ECMO centers has been advocated by The International ECMO Network.
- The process of accepting, retrieving, and successfully transporting a critically ill patient requiring ECMO is a complex endeavor best performed by a specialized ECMO transport team.
- Transport of the most critically ill patients is best performed on ECMO and can be safely performed with careful planning, teamwork, and a highly trained team.

INTRODUCTION

Since the first successful open heart operation using a "heart–lung machine" in 1953, extracorporeal membrane oxygenation (ECMO), or extracorporeal life support, has seen significant technological advances with respect to ECMO cannulas, gas exchange membranes, pumps, and circuit components.[1,2] Since it began collecting data in 1990, the Extracorporeal Life Support Organization (ELSO) registry (**Fig. 1**) has reported 87,366 ECMO runs as of January, 2017, and this rapidly increasing number will undoubtedly continue to grow.[3]

As experience with ECMO continues to evolve, there is growing consensus among experts in the field that it should be performed in "centers with sufficient experience,

[a] Critical Care Medicine, Cooper University Hospital, One Cooper Plaza, D427C, Camden, NJ 08103, USA; [b] Innovative ECMO Concepts, Inc, 13181 Waterrock Lane, Arcadia, OK 73007, USA; [c] Pulmonary Critical Care Sleep Medicine, Fort Belvoir Army Hospital, 9300 DeWitt Loop, FT Belvoir, VA 22060, USA; [d] Uniformed Services University of Health Sciences, 4301 Jones Bridge Road, Bethesda, MD 20814, USA
* Corresponding author. 3106 Burroughs Mill Circle, Cherry Hill, NJ 08002.
E-mail address: niziolkc@gmail.com

Crit Care Clin 33 (2017) 883–896
http://dx.doi.org/10.1016/j.ccc.2017.06.009
0749-0704/17/© 2017 Elsevier Inc. All rights reserved.

Overall Outcomes				
	Total Runs	Survived ECLS		Survived to DC or Transfer
Neonatal				
Pulmonary	26,719	22,394	83%	19,252	72%
Cardiac	7,266	4,727	65%	2,987	41%
ECPR	1,613	1,089	67%	666	41%
Pediatric				
Pulmonary	8,287	5,608	67%	4,812	58%
Cardiac	9,593	6,620	69%	4,941	51%
ECPR	3,615	2,078	57%	1,508	41%
Adult				
Pulmonary	13,712	9,174	66%	8,040	58%
Cardiac	12,566	7,181	57%	5,222	41%
ECPR	3,995	1,572	39%	1,144	28%
Total	87,366	60,443	69%	48,572	55%

Centers

Centers by year

	1990	1991	1992	1993	1994	1995	1996	1997	1998	1999	2000	2001	2002	2003	2004	2005	2006	2007	2008	2009	2010	2011	2012	2013	2014	2015	2016	2017
Centers	83	86	98	111	111	112	115	112	115	111	114	115	119	117	117	129	131	134	140	163	181	200	239	266	303	323	329	251
Cases	1644	1775	1933	1910	1879	1876	1868	1743	1720	1722	1859	1855	1908	1974	1907	2183	2346	2564	2802	3260	3443	4009	5076	6098	7545	8529	9127	2807

Fig. 1. Extracorporeal life support (ECLS) Registry Report International Summary demonstrating increased use of ECLS in adults. DC, discharge; ECPR, extracorporeal cardiopulmonary resuscitation. (*From* ECLS registry report: international summary. 2017; with permission. Available at: www.elso.org. Accessed 24 July, 2017).

volume, and expertise to ensure it is used safely."[4] Thus, the development of ECMO programs has necessitated the formation of ECMO transport teams with the requisite expertise to perform these complex transports.[5] The rapid increase of extracorporeal support in adults has created an increased need for expedient and safe transport of patients on ECMO. A growing body of literature suggests that adult patients can be safely transported on extracorporeal support. Additionally, it is the author's opinion that transport of the most critically ill patients is in fact safer once a patient is placed on extracorporeal support and the literature has begun to suggest this.[6] As the demand for ECMO increases, so will the need for highly specialized teams that can quickly deploy and initiate extracorporeal support in a multiplicity of environments. The purpose of this review is to discuss the state of knowledge with respect to ECMO transport with special emphasis given to how to actually undertake such complex missions.

EVOLUTION OF TRANSPORT WHILE ON EXTRACORPOREAL MEMBRANE OXYGENATION SUPPORT

Cannulating a patient at a referring hospital and transporting on ECMO was first described by Bartlett and colleagues[7] in 1977, who reported 2 transports in their original series of 28 patients. One of their survivors was a 17-year-old patient initiated on venoarterial ECMO and subsequently moved from Albuquerque, New Mexico, to Orange County Medical Center. The team used a US Air Force C-130 and had to hand crank the pump to and from the airfield in the back of a requisitioned bread truck.[8]

As the benefit from ECMO became apparent, particularly in the neonatal and pediatric populations, referrals for ECMO increased. Some of the unique challenges of transporting ECMO patients were described by Boedy and colleagues,[9] who were the first to discuss the hidden mortality of ECMO referral. Boedy reported a mortality of 11% (18 of 158 infants) before leaving the outlying hospital, during transport, or shortly after arrival at their ECMO center over a 52-month period. This and similar experiences at other centers prompted the development of specialized teams and portable ECMO equipment first reported by Cornish and colleagues.[10,11] Nearly 20 years later, despite all transports provided by a dedicated ECMO team, the CESAR trial still reported 3 deaths before transfer and 2 deaths during transfer (one of which was a serious adverse event attributed to mechanical failure of the ambulance's oxygen supply), highlighting the high mortality in this population.[12]

Further driving the increased demand for ECMO transport teams is a increasing body of evidence suggesting that higher volume centers are associated with improved mortality.[13–15] Additionally, data from the influenza A (H1N1) pandemic suggests that the best results were obtained in specialized centers with higher patient numbers and in countries with organized and/or regulated ECMO programs.[2] This led The International ECMO Network to recommend an annual volume of 20 cases per year and that a minimum of 12 of those cases should be performed for acute respiratory failure.[4] To ensure the requisite volume and expertise, The International ECMO Network position statement suggests a "wheel and spoke" model with a network of hospitals created around ECMO referral centers, which will ideally maintain ECMO teams to initiate support, retrieve, and transport patients.[4]

The development of ECMO transport teams has led to a niche area within critical care transport medicine with its own volume of literature. As this area continues to grow, the published experience in ECMO transport varies widely among centers, with only 6 centers reporting more than 100 transports to our knowledge: the University Medical Center at Regensburg, Germany; The Glenfield Hospital, Leicestershire, United Kingdom; the University of Arkansas for Medical Sciences College of Medicine, Little Rock, Arkansas; The University of Michigan, Ann Arbor, Michigan; Columbia University Medical Center, New-York Presbyterian Hospital, New York, New York; and Karolinska University Hospital, Stockholm, Sweden, which has reported more than 845 transports to date.[5,16–21] **Table 1** lists some of the available details regarding the highest volume transport centers.

TRANSPORT LOGISTICS WHILE ON EXTRACORPOREAL MEMBRANE OXYGENATION SUPPORT

The process of accepting, retrieving, and successfully transporting a critically ill patient requiring ECMO support is a complex endeavor, which has been refined and mastered by a growing number of organizations internationally.[16–23] The decision to undertake such a complex mission typically represents the first phase of this process beginning with a referral request to an ECMO capable center. Specific referral criteria may be disseminated to all regional intensive care units to streamline patient selection in a

Table 1
Publications detailing characteristics of large volume ECMO centers

Center	Patients	Age Group	Transport	Distance (Miles)	AE	Reference
Arkansas	112	1 d–69 y	Ground, rotor, fixed wing	Average 250	No deaths Unreported AE	Clement et al,[18] 2010
Columbia	100	Adult Median 40 ± 14.4 y	Ground, fixed wing	2.5–7084	No deaths AE before transport	Biscotti et al,[20] 2015
Leicestershire	102	Adult Mean 41.2 ± 13.1	Ground, rotor, fixed wing	Average 195; range, 3.6–980	No deaths AE before transport	Vaja et al,[17] 2015
Michigan	221	Neonatal, pediatric, adult	Ground, rotor, fixed wing	Average 108 ± 122	1 death	Bryner et al,[19] 2014
Stockholm	322[a]	Neonatal, pediatric, adult	Ground, rotor, fixed wing	4.3–8357	No deaths AE reported	Broman et al,[21] 2015
Regensberg	>180	NR	NR	NR	NR	Lunz et al,[16] 2013

[a] To date has performed over 845 transports.[5]
Abbreviations: AE, adverse events; ECMO, extracorporeal membrane oxygenation; NR, not reported.

centralized health system and/or considered on a case-by-case basis.[22,23] Depending on the referral, the transport may be defined as a primary or secondary transport. Primary transports are situations where the transport team performs cannulation at the referring facility and transports the patient to an ECMO center, whereas secondary transports are situations where the patient has already been cannulated, but requires transfer to another facility.[24] Once a patient has been accepted as a potential ECMO candidate, the ECMO team is mobilized and mission planning begins based on the specific situation.

MISSION PLANNING

When a transport request is accepted the transport team's number one priority must be patient and team safety, and all preparations should be made with this in mind. Additionally, a second priority according to the ELSO transport guidelines is expediting team arrival at the referral facility for primary transports, because this timing could be potentially life saving; however, this factor may not be as critical for secondary transports (when a patient has already been cannulated).[24] It is also important to maintain close communication with the referring facility before and during team transport.

For example, a second ECMO coordinator at the Arkansas Children's Hospital maintains communication with the referring hospital once the team is en route, relaying instructions regarding surgical space and equipment, availability of family members for consent, and arrangement of blood products. Additionally, the coordinator arranges for temporary medical privileges for the transport team.[22] To bypass this requirement, The University of Michigan legal department has developed an "umbrella policy" signed by the referring physician upon arrival, essentially transferring full responsibility of the patient to the ECMO transport team, thus allowing them to act as though they were practicing at their own institution.[25] Additionally, the ECMO team must consider the mode of transportation, equipment requirements, and team composition necessary to complete the mission.

MODE OF TRANSPORT

The distance between the ECMO center and outlying hospital as well as weather conditions are both major factors in determining the best mode of transport. Additionally, some programs will only have access to ground transportation, whereas others will use a combination of ground, rotor, and fixed wing aircraft.[17–19,21,23,26] Depending on the available resources, some programs will use dedicated transport platforms such as a dedicated ECMO ambulance, whereas other programs have developed streamlined protocols relying on the local ambulance system.[17,26]

According to ELSO guidelines, if the duration of en route care is expected to exceed 3 to 4 hours by ground, then air transport should be considered. General distance references are ground transport for 250 miles (400 km) or less, helicopters for 400 miles (650 km) or less, and fixed wing aircraft for missions of more than 400 miles (650 km). Additionally, weather conditions such as poor visibility and cloud cover may preclude the use of certain modes of transport. For example, medical helicopters and fixed wing aircraft are frequently not capable of instrument flight rules flight. Instrument flight rules flight enables flight in poor weather conditions, such as low visibility and cloud cover, but requires additional specialized pilot training, navigation equipment, and flight planning with air traffic control not normally required for visual flight rules, or navigation by sight. This condition may necessitate ground transport, depending on patient acuity and the need for immediate transport, even though air transport would have normally been preferred. **Table 2** details the capabilities of ground ambulances, helicopters, and fixed wing transport from the ELSO guidelines for ECMO transport.[24]

Table 2 Aircraft and vehicle capabilities			
	Ground Ambulance	**Helicopter**	**Fixed Wing Aircraft**
Space for team and equipment	Sufficient (4–5 team members)	More limited (3–5 team members)	Variable ($\geq$4 team members)
Noise	Relatively little	Very loud	Loud
Distance range for reasonable transport times	Up to 250–300 miles (400 km)	Up to 300–400 miles (650 km)	Any distance
Weight limitations	Unlimited	Limited (impacted by distance and weather)	Variable (depending on aircraft and conditions)
Loading and securing equipment and ECMO circuit and patient	Relatively easy	Relatively easy	Variable (depending on equipment and aircraft model)
Cost	++	+++	++++

Abbreviation: ECMO, extracorporeal membrane oxygenation.

From Extracorporeal Life Support Organization (ELSO). 2015. Guidelines for ECMO Transport; with permission. Available at: https://www.elso.org/resources/guidelines.aspx. Accessed 15 March, 2017.

EQUIPMENT

In theory, the equipment required during an ECMO transport mission is the same equipment used while caring for a patient in the hospital; however, the out-of-hospital environment poses unique challenges requiring careful planning and special modification. Once the transport team embarks on a mission, it must be a self-contained unit with patient survival ultimately depending on the team's ability to troubleshoot and manage complications en route. As a result, the team must travel with a comprehensive armamentarium of supplies; however, size and weight constraints of the transport platform typically limit what the team can transport. As a result, careful selection of equipment is pivotal with appropriate back-up supplies as necessary.

As technology has evolved, centrifugal pumps permitting shorter circuit length and miniaturization of transport monitors have decreased the size and weight of equipment that must be transported.[8] Cornish and colleagues[11] first used a Rubbermaid Healthcare Utility Cart modified with aluminum cross-braces with an Ohio transport isolette and military litter secured on top. Since that time, transport sleds as well as ECMO systems have been designed specifically for ECMO transport. Lunz and colleagues[16] have reported the successful air transport of patients on the Deltastream DP3 in venovenous ECMO, a miniaturized light-weight ECMO system weighing only 5 kg. With these significant improvements, it is important to note that all equipment used for air transport must meet airworthiness standards established by relevant regulatory agencies such as the Federal Aviation Administration to ensure the equipment can safely function in flight and its electromagnetic interference does not compromise flight operations.[24]

In addition to the ECMO circuit, stretcher or sled device, and necessary monitors, the ECMO team must ensure there is a power source capable of sustaining critical equipment for transport to and from the transport platform and in the event of vehicle or aircraft power failure. There should also be a sufficient supply of oxygen as well as all necessary medications and additional medical supplies with back-up ECMO circuits, ventilator tubing, and other mission critical supplies. Blood products are usually provided by the referring facility and should be arranged in advance. Most important, all equipment should be inspected before departure and the ELSO guidelines recommend completion of a checklist to ensure all critical items are present and functioning.[24] The importance of using a checklist and testing critical items cannot be overstated.

TEAM COMPOSITION

Depending on the institution, the ECMO transport team typically consists of a combination of intensivists, surgeons, nurses, respiratory therapists, ECMO specialists, and emergency medical services providers. Team composition may need to be adjusted depending on the clinical scenario, for example, whether or not a patient requires cannulation or additional personnel required for long distance transports. Regardless of team composition, there should be a designated medical director or mission commander responsible for the transport team and safe transport of the patient, as well as a physician with significant ECMO experience and an ECMO specialist to manage the circuit.[8,24]

Team composition among centers reporting more than 100 transports is as follows. The Arkansas Children's Hospital team typically consists of an ECMO coordinator, pediatric cardiac surgeon, surgical assistant, and intensive care physician.[18] The Columbia University Medical Center team consists of a cardiothoracic surgeon, surgical fellow, 2 perfusionists, and 2 critical care paramedics.[20] The Glenfield Hospital uses a role-specific team, including someone with training in cannulation, intensive care, perfusion, and an ECMO specialist nurse.[17] The University of Michigan cannulation team consists of a critical care surgeon, a critical care fellow, 2 flight nurses, and 2 ECMO specialists.[19] Stockholm, which has reported the most transports in the literature, uses an ECMO physician (anesthetist and team leader), intensive care nurse, cannulating surgeon, and occasionally a scrub nurse for primary cannulation.[21] The Regensberg team consists of a cardiac anesthesiologist and a clinical perfusionist.[16]

FLIGHT CONSIDERATIONS

Higher flight altitudes decrease transport time, turbulence, and fuel consumption; however, specific attention should be given to the flight environment's effect on patient care as well as the ECMO circuit.[24] Specifically, the aviation environment leads to unique considerations with respect to atmospheric pressure, oxygenation, temperature, noise and vibration, acceleration and deceleration forces, humidity, and vision.[27–29] **Box 1** shows some of the common changes of flight and their potential adverse effects.

Atmospheric Pressure

Modern jet aircraft typically fly at cruising altitudes ranging from 28,000 to 43,000 feet. Atmospheric pressure decreases with increasing altitude from 760 mm Hg (14.7 psi) at sea level to 176 mm Hg (3.4 psi) at 35,000 feet.[30] According to Boyle's law, as the pressure of a confined gas decreases, the volume of that gas will increase inversely.[31] This principle results in the expansion of gas in air-filled organs such as lungs, intestines, and sinuses, which can lead to symptoms such as ear pain, sinus pain, tooth pain, and abdominal pain until the gas is released.[27,28] More seriously, gas expansion can lead to more life-threatening adverse effects such as expansion of a previously stable pneumothorax.[31] As a result, airplane cabins are pressurized to lower levels; however, this is rarely equalized to sea level.[30] Hampson and colleagues[32] used a handheld mountaineering altimeter carried on 207 flights aboard 17 different aircraft and noted that the average peak cabin altitude was 6341 ± 1813 feet. Thus, medical

Box 1
Changes in flight and impact on patient transport

Changes in Flight	Adverse Effects
Decreased atmospheric pressure	Trapped gas
	• Ear pain
	• Sinus pain
	• Abdominal pain
	• Tooth pain
	Expansion of pneumothorax
Decreased partial pressure of oxygen	Hypoxia
Decreased temperature	Hypothermia
Noise	Hearing loss
	Communication difficulty
	Missed alarms
Vibration	Dislodgement of lines or tubes
Acceleration and deceleration forces	Unwanted patient movement
	Medical devices as projectiles
Decreased humidity	Dehydration
Visual impairment	Spatial disorientation

crews should be aware of these effects and ensure tubes such as chest tubes and nasogastric tubes are vented.

Oxygenation

As altitude increases, the partial pressure of oxygen also decreases along with pressure. At sea level, the partial pressure of alveolar oxygen is normally 107 mm Hg, but decreases to 59 mm Hg at an altitude of 7500 to 8000 feet.[31] At an altitude of 45,000 feet, a human rapidly exposed to the atmosphere would be unconscious in 9 to 12 seconds with death following shortly thereafter.[28] Even with a pressurized cabin, there is still a decrease in the partial pressure of alveolar oxygen, which can lead to obvious consequences for a patient with already severe underlying cardiovascular compromise. Specifically for a patient on ECMO, the team should anticipate decreased gas exchange capability of the membrane oxygenator with reduced atmospheric pressure. With a cabin pressure of 6900 feet, an oxygenator requires an Fio_2 of 1 to achieve the same capacity of an Fio_2 of 0.8 at sea level. In an unpressurized helicopter at less than 5000 feet, a decrease of oxygen saturation (SpO_2) by 3% to 4% should be anticipated.[8] **Fig. 2** illustrates altitudes effect on the oxyhemoglobin dissociation curve.

Temperature

With increasing height above sea level, the temperature drops by 3.6°F (2°C) for every 1000 feet of ascent, which is referred to as the lapse rate.[27]

Noise and Vibration

Engine noise leads to communication difficulties between crew members and alarms might not be heard.[33] Vibration and subsequent patient movement, especially on take-off and landing, risk disruption of tubing connections and indwelling line placement.

Acceleration and Deceleration Forces

The transport team must ensure the patient and all equipment is appropriately secured to prevent medical equipment from becoming dangerous projectiles.

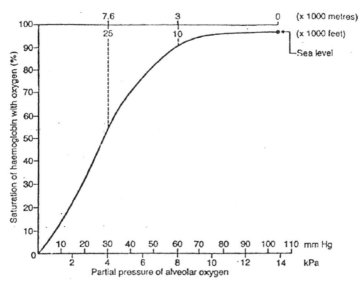

Fig. 2. Oxyhemoglobin dissociation curve. (*Data from* Aerospace Medical Association. Medical guidelines of airline travel stresses of flight. 2014. Available at: www.asma.org/asma/media/asma/Travel-Publications/Medical%20Guidelines/Stresses-of-Flight-Nov-2014.pdf. Accessed 15 March, 2017.)

Humidity

Aircraft inevitably have low cabin humidity ranging from 10% to 20% because the outside air at high altitude is essentially devoid of moisture. More important for long flights, dry air necessitates appropriate fluid intake to prevent dehydration and the medical team must account for this by staying well-hydrated and being mindful of hypovolemia in their patient.[29]

Vision

Vision is the first of the body's special senses to be affected by lack of oxygen and impairment can be detected at altitudes of 5000 feet at nighttime and 10,000 feet during the day.[28]

ADVERSE EVENTS

Extracorporeal support is a highly specialized treatment modality with complications such as catheter site hemorrhage, surgical site hemorrhage, pneumothorax, and catheter-related infection well-documented in the literature.[34] In addition to the host of complications pertaining to extracorporeal support, the inherent nature of transporting such a critically ill patient on multiple different life support devices adds an additional layer of complexity and opportunity for error or adverse events.

Ericsson and colleagues[5] recently published a retrospective descriptive analysis of 514 ECMO transports conducted by their group from January 2010 to June 2016 for which medical records could be identified that specifically examined adverse events. In their single-center series, 206 adverse events occurred in 163 transports (31.6%). Sixty-five percent of the adverse events were classified as patient related, most

---

Box 2
Transport complications and their prevention and management

Complication	Prevention and Management
Hypoxia	• Optimize mechanical ventilation (increase PEEP or Fio_2) • Increase blood flow rate on ECMO circuit • Transfuse blood products to correct anemia
Hypotension	• Perform a complete ECMO circuit check (ensure no cannula kinking or dislodgement) • Increase flow and sweep gas rates • Use ultrasound imaging as available to assess for pneumothorax or pericardial tamponade and treat as indicated • Treat hypovolemia with blood products or crystalloids or colloids • Initiate vasopressors or inotropes as indicated
Delayed pneumothorax	• Carefully review all imaging before departure • Tube thoracostomy insertion
Line or tube dislodgement	• Check position of all lines and tubes before departure • If cannula dislodgment, support hemodynamics and proceed to closest appropriate location for reinsertion • Replace as needed
Power failure	• Ensure maximum charge of all equipment • Transport with back-up power source

Abbreviations: ECMO, extracorporeal membrane oxygenation; PEEP, positive end-expiratory pressure.

---

commonly loss of tidal volume and pulmonary edema (43%). Less common were adverse events related to equipment (14.6%), staff (5.8%), vehicle (12.6%), and environmental (1.9%) factors, such as freezing of intravenous lines and stopcocks. In their series, 7.8% of adverse events were classified as an immediate threat to life with equipment and technical complications being most common (ie, clotting of the ECMO circuit). There were no reported deaths. **Box 2** details common complications encountered while transporting patient's on ECMO with prevention and management strategies.

A recent systematic review published by Mendes and colleagues[6] included a total of 38 articles and 1481 patients (1025 adult, 456 pediatric) and examined complications and mortality of patients transported on ECMO. Overall survival rates were 62% (95% CI, 57–68) for adults and 68% (95% CI, 60–75) for pediatric patients, which is congruent with published ELSO data demonstrating no increase in mortality for ECMO support despite the need for transport to a referral center.[6] At least 1 complication was reported in 12 of the analyzed articles, totaling 80 occurrences with 2 reported deaths with a transport mortality rate of 0.1%. This is in contrast with the CESAR trial, with patients transported by an ECMO team without ECMO support during transport and 2 of 90 patients dying during transport with a transport mortality rate of 2%.[12] The authors go on to suggest that a strategy of rapid ECMO initiation and transfer may be safer.[6] Although there has been no study specifically examining whether transport on ECMO affects mortality to our knowledge, it is the opinion of these authors that rapid cannulation by a highly trained ECMO team followed by transport to an ECMO center is preferred and can be done safely.

SUMMARY

The rapid increase of extracorporeal support for severe acute respiratory failure as well as evidence suggesting high-volume ECMO centers have improved

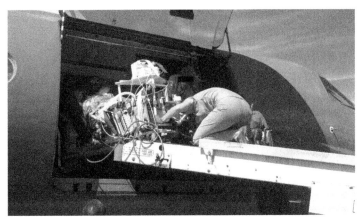

Fig. 3. Loading patient for transport using a conveyer belt.

outcomes has created an increased need for the expedient and safe transport of patients on ECMO. The process of accepting, retrieving, and successfully transporting a critically ill patient requiring ECMO is a complex endeavor with an increase number of centers developing ECMO transport programs. The out-of-hospital environment poses unique challenges, but multiple high-volume centers have demonstrated that specialized transport teams can successfully transport patients on ECMO. Although adverse events can occur, death is rare, and cannulating a patient before transport and transporting on ECMO may in fact be safer than transporting a patient to a referral center for cannulation (**Figs. 3–5**).

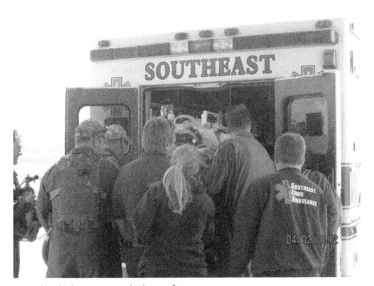

Fig. 4. Patient loaded into an ambulance for transport.

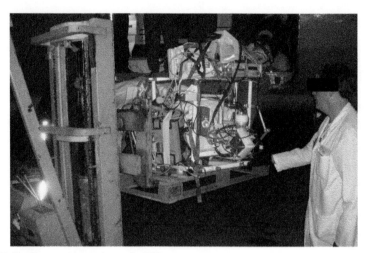

Fig. 5. Unloading patient using a forklift.

REFERENCES

1. Gibbon J. Development of the artificial heart and lung extracorporeal blood circuit. JAMA 1968;206(9):1983–6.

2. Schmidt M, Hodgson C, Combes A. Extracorporeal gas exchange for acute respiratory failure in adult patients: a systematic review. Crit Care 2015;19:99.

3. Extracorporeal Life Support Organization (ELSO). ECLS Registry Report International Summary. Available at: https://www.elso.org/Registry/Statistics/Interna tionalSummary.aspx. Accessed 15 March, 2017.

4. Combes A, Brodie D, Barlett R, et al. Position paper for the organization of extracorporeal membrane oxygenation programs for acute respiratory failure in adult patients. Am J Respir Crit Care Med 2014;190:488–96.

5. Ericsson A, Frenckner B, Broman LM. Adverse events during inter-hospital transports on extracorporeal membrane oxygenation. Prehosp Emerg Care 2017; 21(4):448–55.

6. Mendes PV, de Albuquerque Gallo C, Besen BA, et al. Transportation of patients on extracorporeal membrane oxygenation: a tertiary medical center experience and systematic review of the literature. Ann Intensive Care 2017;7(1):14.

7. Bartlett RH, Gazzaniga AB, Fong SW, et al. Extracorporeal membrane oxygenator support for cardiopulmonary failure. Experience in 28 cases. J Thorac Cardiovasc Surg 1977;73:375–86.

8. Cannon JW, Allan PF, Phillip A, et al. Inter-hospital transport of the ECMO patient from concept to implementation. In: Annich GM, Lynch WR, MacLauren G, et al, editors. ECMO: extracorporeal cardiopulmonary support in critical care. 4th edition. Ann Arbor (MI): Extracorporeal Life Support Organization; 2012.

9. Boedy RF, Howell CG, Kanto WP Jr. Hidden mortality rate associated with extracorporeal membrane oxygenation. J Pediatr 1990;117:462–4.

10. Cornish JD, Gerstmann DR, Begnaud MJ, et al. Inflight use of extracorporeal membrane oxygenation for severe neonatal respiratory failure. Perfusion 1986; 1:281–7.

11. Cornish JD, Carter JM, Gerstmann DR, et al. Extracorporeal membrane oxygenation as a means of stabilizing and transporting high risk neonates. ASAIO Trans 1991;37(4):564.

12. Peek GJ, Mugford M, Tiruvoipati R, et al. CESAR trial collaboration. Efficacy and economic assessment of conventional ventilatory support versus extracorporeal membrane oxygenation for severe adult respiratory failure (CESAR): a multicentre randomised controlled trial. Lancet 2009;374(9698):1351–63.

13. Karamlou T, Vafaeezadeh M, Parrish AM, et al. Increased extracorporeal membrane oxygenation center case volume is associated with improved extracorporeal membrane oxygenation survival among pediatric patients. J Thorac Cardiovasc Surg 2013;145(2):470–5.

14. Freeman CL, Bennett TD, Casper TC, et al. Pediatric and neonatal extracorporeal membrane oxygenation: does center volume impact mortality? Crit Care Med 2014;42(3):512–9.

15. Barbaro RP, Odetola FO, Kidwell KM, et al. Association of hospital-level volume of extracorporeal membrane oxygenation cases and mortality. Analysis of the Extracorporeal Life Support Organization registry. Am J Respir Crit Care Med 2015; 191(8):894–901.

16. Lunz D, Philipp A, Judemann K, et al. First experience with the Deltastream(R) DP3 in venovenous extracorporeal membrane oxygenation and air-supported inter-hospital transport. Interact Cardiovasc Thorac Surg 2013;17(5):773–7.

17. Vaja R, Chauhan I, Joshi V, et al. Five-year experience with mobile adult extracorporeal membrane oxygenation in a tertiary referral center. J Crit Care 2015;30(6): 1195–8.

18. Clement KC, Fiser RT, Fiser WP, et al. Single-institution experience with interhospital extracorporeal membrane oxygenation transport: a descriptive study. Pediatr Crit Care Med 2010;11(4):509–13.

19. Bryner B, Cooley E, Copenhaver W, et al. Two decades' experience with interfacility transport on extracorporeal membrane oxygenation. Ann Thorac Surg 2014; 98(4):1363–70.

20. Biscotti M, Agerstrand C, Abrams D, et al. One hundred transports on extracorporeal support to an extracorporeal membrane oxygenation center. Ann Thorac Surg 2015;100(1):34–9 [discussion: 39–40].

21. Broman LM, Holzgraefe B, Palmér K, et al. The Stockholm experience: interhospital transports on extracorporeal membrane oxygenation. Crit Care 2015;19:278.

22. Cabrera AG, Prodhan P, Cleves MA, et al. Interhospital transport of children requiring extracorporeal membrane oxygenation support for cardiac dysfunction. Congenit Heart Dis 2011;6(3):202–8.

23. Forrest P, Ratchford J, Burns B, et al. Retrieval of critically ill adults using extracorporeal membrane oxygenation: an Australian experience. Intensive Care Med 2011;37(5):824–30.

24. Extracorporeal Life Support Organization (ELSO). 2015. Guidelines for ECMO Transport. Available at: https://www.elso.org/resources/guidelines.aspx. Accessed 15 March, 2017.

25. Foley DS, Pranikoff T, Younger JG, et al. A review of 100 patients transported on extracorporeal life support. ASAIO J 2002;48(6):612–9.

26. Yeo HJ, Cho WH, Park JM, et al. Interhospital transport system for critically ill patients: mobile extracorporeal membrane oxygenation without a ventilator. Korean J Thorac Cardiovasc Surg 2017;50(1):8–13.

27. DeHart RL. Health issues of air travel. Annu Rev Public Health 2003;24:133–51.

28. Federal Aviation Administration (FAA). Introduction to aviation physiology. Available at: https://www.faa.gov/pilots/training/airman_education/media/IntroAviationPhys. pdf. Accessed 15 March, 2017.

29. Aerospace Medical Association (ASMA). Medical guidelines of airline travel stresses of flight. 2014. Available at: https://www.asma.org/asma/media/asma/ Travel-Publications/Medical%20Guidelines/Stresses-of-Flight-Nov-2014.pdf. Accessed 15 March, 2017.

30. AMA commission on emergency medical services: medical aspects of transportation aboard commercial aircraft. JAMA 1982;247:1007–11.

31. Bunch A, Duchateau FX, Verner L, et al. Commercial air travel after pneumothorax: a review of the literature. Air Med J 2013;32(5):268–74.

32. Hampson NB, Kregenow DA, Mahoney AM, et al. Altitude exposures during commercial flight: a reappraisal. Aviat Space Environ Med 2013;84(1):27–31.

33. Broman LM, Frenckner B. Transportation of critically ill patients on extracorporeal membrane oxygenation. Front Pediatr 2016;4:63.

34. Bhatt N, Osborn E. Extracorporeal gas exchange: the expanding role of extracorporeal support in respiratory failure. Clin Chest Med 2016;37:765–80.

Medication Complications in Extracorporeal Membrane Oxygenation

Ami G. Shah, PharmD[a],*, Michelle Peahota, PharmD[a],
Brandi N. Thoma, PharmD[a], Walter K. Kraft, MD[b]

KEYWORDS

- Pharmacology • Pharmacokinetics • Therapeutic drug monitoring

KEY POINTS

- Extracorporeal membrane oxygenation (ECMO) is associated with physiologic and biomechanical changes that can impact drug disposition.
- There are limited data describing changes in drug pharmacokinetic parameters for patients treated with ECMO.
- Changes in pharmacokinetics are often drug specific.
- Extrapolation of ECMO data from neonatal literature is limited due to significant differences in body composition and elimination pathways.
- Therapeutic drug monitoring, when possible, should be considered to individualize therapeutics in patients receiving ECMO therapy.

INTRODUCTION

Critically ill patients have alterations in the pharmacokinetic (PK) parameters that describe drug absorption, distribution, metabolism, and excretion. These disturbances arise from the acute response of critical illness, including systemic inflammatory responses, organ dysfunction, altered tissue permeability, pH disturbances, changes in intravascular or extravascular space, fluid shifts, or decreased protein concentration. These PK alterations are relevant, as they may precipitate unexpected medication toxicities or impair efficacy. To optimize patient outcomes, PK changes should be as best possible identified when developing medication regimens for critically ill patients.[1–4]

a Department of Pharmacy, Thomas Jefferson University Hospital, 111 South 11th Street, Suite 2260, Philadelphia, PA 19107, USA; b Department of Pharmacology and Experimental Therapeutics, Thomas Jefferson University, 111 South 11th Street, Philadelphia, PA 19107, USA
* Corresponding author. 111 South 11th Street, Suite 2260, Philadelphia, PA 19107.
E-mail address: amishah1221@gmail.com

Crit Care Clin 33 (2017) 897–920
http://dx.doi.org/10.1016/j.ccc.2017.06.010   criticalcare.theclinics.com
0749-0704/17/Published by Elsevier Inc.

EXTRACORPOREAL MEMBRANE OXYGENATION AND PHARMACOKINETICS

Mechanical ventilation, renal replacement therapy (RRT), and extracorporeal membrane oxygenation (ECMO)[5-8] can impact drug disposition and complicate the management of critically ill patients. During ECMO therapy, a large volume of blood is extracted from the venous system and is circulated outside the body into an oxygenator (**Fig. 1**). A typical ECMO circuit consists of polyvinyl chloride (PVC) tubing, a hollow fiber (polymethylpentene) oxygenator, and a heat exchanger.[9] PK changes during critical illness are often more pronounced in the presence of ECMO. Several aspects, such as the sequestration of medications in the ECMO circuit, increased volume of distribution, and alterations in organ perfusion may alter PK parameters in patients receiving ECMO[5,7,9-12] (**Table 1**).

The effect of ECMO therapy on PK varies and is not fully elucidated for most drugs. Investigating the impact of the ECMO circuit and its resulting physiologic changes on PK and pharmacodynamics (PD) is difficult given the limited patient population on which to generate data. The ECMO population is numbered because ECMO is often a salvage therapy offered by limited number of centers. The available data investigating ECMO therapy is not only limited in size, but is typically also observational because it is difficult to conduct randomized trials with a control group. Although there is some literature available in neonatal populations, it is difficult to generalize these data to adult populations. ECMO technology is frequently evolving, and circuits' manufacturers and materials vary, further limiting data generalizability. Demands of clinical care and blood volume during critical illness make sparse PK sampling with population modeling methods the only feasible method to investigate drug PK parameters in these patients. Although this approach can identify some covariates associated with differential drug disposition, it is not possible to generate precise PK parameters under a variety of clinical scenarios.

ECMO Circuit

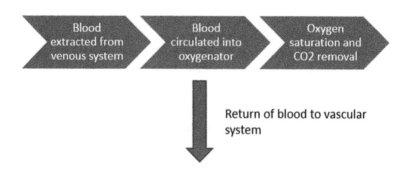

Fig. 1. ECMO configuration.

Table 1
Pharmacokinetic changes in critically ill patients

Pharmacokinetic Parameter	Observed Physiologic Changes in Critically Ill Patients	Resultant Pharmacokinetic Changes
Absorption	• Decreased gastrointestinal and subcutaneous perfusion	• Decreased time to peak concentration and area under the curve
Distribution	• Decreased albumin • Decrease tissue and organ perfusion	• Increased free drug concentration and volumes of distribution for albumin-bound medications • Increased volumes of distribution for hydrophilic medications • Reduced free drug concentrations in peripheral tissues
Metabolism	• Acute reduction in hepatic blood flow • Alteration of hepatic enzyme function	• Reduced clearance of hepatically cleared medications
Elimination	• Acute kidney insufficiency • Alteration of active transport of medications	• Reduced clearance of renally cleared medications

Data from Smith BS, Yogaratnam D, Levasseur-Franklin KE, et al. Introduction to drug pharmacokinetics in the critically Ill patient. Chest 2012;141(5):1327–36.

Drug Sequestration

Drug sequestration to the circuit is a common consequence of ECMO therapy. The loss of medication in the circuit depends on factors including surface area or the potential interaction of medications to various plastic components of the ECMO system.[5] The type of circuit may also be a variable predictor influencing the level of drug sequestration.[9,13,14] The presence and material of ECMO oxygenators may further result in drug recovery differences.[15,16] The use of blood versus crystalloid priming agents may increase drug losses with specific medications, such as fosphenytoin, fentanyl, and heparin.[9,11,17] The overall effect of priming ECMO circuits with crystalloids, colloids, or blood products on drug sequestration is poorly characterized. Although saline is a commonly used priming agent for ECMO circuits, there is currently no standard recommendation or guidance surrounding the most optimal priming approach. Molecular drug properties, such as lipophilicity, molecular size, ionization, and protein binding, characteristically influence the likelihood of drug sequestration in the ECMO circuit. Typically, lipophilic and highly protein-bound medications are significantly sequestered in the circuit.[9,18] PK parameters of hydrophilic medications also are affected secondary to hemodilution and other ECMO-related pathophysiologic changes. Previous studies investigating the overall impact of drug sequestration have reported up to 50% of morphine and 40% of lorazepam sequestration at 24 hours with additional medication losses in older circuits.[17] Most importantly, the sequestration phenomenon is unpredictable. Although medications may be sequestered, the circuit also may continue to release the sequestrated product over time. Overall, the sequestration of medications in the ECMO circuit increases the volume of distribution (Vd), which ultimately causes lower or suboptimal drug concentrations in the body (**Table 2**).

Volume of Distribution

Vd is the hypothetical body space available for the medication to be diluted and distributed. Conceptually, Vd can be thought of as the relative fraction of drug that

Table 2	
Impact of extracorporeal membrane oxygenation on drug pharmacokinetics	
Change in PK Parameter	**Relating Factor**
↑ Vd	Priming of tubing
	Hemodilution
	Drug sequestration within tubing/circuit
	SIRS/Sepsis
	Organ failure
	Hydrophilicity of drug
↑ Cl	SIRS/Sepsis
	Drug inactivation within circuit
↓ Cl	Organ failure
↑↓ Cl	Hydrophilicity of drug[a]
	Lipophilicity of drug[b]
↓ Cmax	Priming of tubing
	Hemodilution
	Drug sequestration within tubing/circuit
	Hydrophilicity of drug

Abbreviations: ↑, increase; ↓, decrease; Cl, clearance; Cmax, maximum concentration; PK, pharmacokinetic; SIRS, systemic inflammatory response syndrome; Vd, volume of distribution.
[a] Dependent on renal function.
[b] Dependent on hepatic function.

resides within the blood volume compared with that sequestered in extravascular compartments. Volume status and medication volume of distribution are highly relevant when predicting effective medication dosages for patients. Drug concentrations are measured in the central compartment and in variable fashion is a proxy for drug concentration at target, and thus drug effect. The therapeutic impact of an altered Vd is highest with medications with small volumes of distribution. For example, gentamicin is an aminoglycoside with a relatively small Vd of 0.2 to 0.3 L/kg in healthy adults, or 18 L in an average 70-kg patient. A typical initial 2 mg/kg dose in this patient would lead to approximate therapeutic concentrations of 140 mg/18 L, or 8 mg/L. The target peak concentration of conventionally dosed gentamicin in severe gram-negative infections is 8 to 10 mg/L. Even slight changes in Vd may have a drastic impact on plasma concentrations. For example, the final concentration would be subtherapeutic at 5 mg/L if the Vd were increased to 0.4 L/kg (28 L) or supratherapeutic at 20 mg/L if the Vd were decreased to 0.1 L/kg (7 L). In contrast, medications that have a large Vd have the ability to diffuse from tissue reservoirs back into the circulating plasma. Unlike distribution to extravascular tissue, drug sequestered in tubing will not redistribute into the system when tubing is replaced. Other mechanisms by which ECMO has been found to increase Vd include changes in plasma proteins from hemodilution or transfusions, organ dysfunction, pH alterations, and the activation of the systematic inflammatory response system. Most PK data in patients receiving ECMO have originated from neonatal populations and in comparison to adults, neonates have a higher proportion of total body water, resulting in a higher Vd for hydrophilic medications. Additionally, neonates have decreased plasma protein binding, trapping less drug in the central compartment and resulting in a higher Vd for protein-bound medications. These differences between adult and neonatal populations limit the applicability of available ECMO PK data across the continuum of ages.[5,11,19,20]

Metabolism and excretion play significant roles in determining optimal medication dosages. A challenge often seen in patients receiving ECMO involves changes in the rates of blood flow, which may alter tissue and organ perfusion.[5] Kidney and liver hypoperfusion can impair medication metabolism and clearance, leading to accumulation and, potentially, toxicity. Renal dysfunction (serum creatinine >1.5 mg/dL), a common occurrence during ECMO, has been reported to be as high as 32% in venovenous (VV) ECMO and 47% in venoarterial (VA) ECMO.[21] Although VV ECMO uses pulsatile blood flow, VA ECMO incorporates higher flow rates with nonpulsatile blood flow. The mode disrupts typical blood flow because the kidneys interpret it as hypotension, causing a downstream activation of the renin-angiotensin system (RASS), ultimately leading to reduced urine production, an increased circulating volume, and thus an increased Vd.[5,19] Much of the available PK data on ECMO have been reported in neonatal populations that typically have immature enzymatic pathways and glomerular function. The impact of blood flow rates and hypoperfusion are yet to be described in the adult populations. Although the impact of renal hypoperfusion may be countered with the use of RRT, the PK of patients on RRT receiving ECMO is complex and variable. Therapeutic drug monitoring, whenever possible, is essential in this patient population. Additional research in this subset of patients is necessary to further guide treatment goals.

Sedation, analgesia, anticoagulation, and treatment of infection are commonly encountered and are areas of concern in patients receiving ECMO. Many medications from these classes have highly variable PK parameters that are unpredictable and patient dependent. Although some medication classes, such vasopressors and other cardioactive drugs, can be titrated to patient response, others, such as sedatives, have nonstandardized endpoint measures. Others have no readily available biomarkers to follow, requiring in all cases the application of PK principles to achieve optimal therapeutic response[22,23] **(Table 3)**.

SEDATIVES/ANALGESICS-OPIOIDS

Sedatives and analgesics are used extensively in the ECMO population. Optimal sedation regimens are poorly defined due to interpatient PK variability. The optimal sedative and analgesic agent depends on multiple PK considerations and patient-specific variables.[24–26] In addition, there is a lack of a well-accepted PD endpoints to allow characterization of exposure/response relationships. Clinically, subjective agitation and ventilator dyssynchrony are common measures of adequacy of sedation. Opioids are commonly used in the intensive care unit (ICU), as they provide both analgesia and sedation. The intravenous (IV) route of administration bypasses concerns for erratic absorption and also allows for faster onset and rapid titratability.[27,28] Although all full mu-agonist opioids can achieve equal levels of analgesia, each agent's potency and physiochemical characteristics serve as differentiating factors.

Fentanyl

Fentanyl, a lipophilic synthetic mu-opioid agonist with rapid onset and a short half-life, has been found to bind to the ECMO circuit extensively after 24 hours.[5,29] The level of fentanyl membrane absorption has been found to be variable dependent on the type of membrane oxygenator.[13] Thus, fentanyl may be suitable for short-term analgesia; however, higher doses may be necessary to provide adequate sedation and analgesia, dependent on the type of membrane oxygenator beyond 24 hours.[5,28] In contrast, the concentrations of morphine, a full mu-opioid agonist, are maintained despite ECMO therapy. Its minimal absorption to the ECMO circuit is likely due to

Table 3
Dosing recommendations

Medication	Standard Dosing Recommendations in Critically Ill Patients	Summary of Recommendations in ECMO	Dosing Recommendations for Patients on ECMO Therapy
Sedatives/analgesics: opioids			
Fentanyl	• 0.35–0.5 mcg/kg IVP q 0.5–1 h intermittent dosing • 0.7–10 mcg/kg/hr infusion	• Higher doses may be necessary to provide adequate sedation and analgesia beyond 24 h	May need to increase rates of fentanyl infusion beyond 24 h; titrate to clinical effect
Morphine	• 2–4 mg IVP q 1–2 h intermittent dosing • 2–30 mg/h infusion	• Concentrations maintained despite ECMO therapy • Clearance of morphine decreases up to 50% potentially due to hepatic hypoperfusion	Decrease rate of morphine infusion and titrate to clinical effect
Hydromorphone	• 0.2–0.6 mg IVP q 1–2 h intermittent dosing • 0.5–3 mg/h infusion	• No studies investigating its pharmacokinetics in ECMO • Hydromorphone is hydrophilic, which is expected to minimize sequestration in ECMO circuit	Standard dosing recommendations
Meperidine	The American Pain Society (2008) and Institute for Safe Medication Practices (2007) do not recommend meperidine's use as an analgesic; if used in acute pain (in patients without renal or CNS disease) cannot be avoided, treatment should be limited to ≤48 h and doses should not exceed 600 mg/24 h	• Commonly avoided due to its potential for drug interactions with serotonergic and dopaminergic agents and metabolite accumulation leading to decreased seizure thresholds	Avoid use
Sedatives/analgesics: NMDA antagonists			
Ketamine	• Bolus: 0.1–0.5 mg/kg • Infusion: 0.05–0.4 mg/kg/h	• In studies, median ketamine doses ranged from 50–100 mg/h	Higher doses may be required; titrate to clinical effect

Sedatives/analgesics: benzodiazepines		
Lorazepam	• LD: 0.02–0.04 mg/kg ($\leq$ 2mg) • MD: 0.02–0.06 mg/kg q2–6 h prn or 0.01–0.1 mg/kg/h ($\leq$10 mg/h)	Lesser degree of ECMO circuit sequestration	Standard dosing recommendations
Midazolam	• LD: 0.01–0.05 mg/kg over several minutes • MD: 0.02–0.1 mg/kg/h	• >50% of midazolam may be sequestered (up to 95% in the first few hours of ECMO initiation) • Accumulation of midazolam's active metabolite or liver and renal failure prolongs the effect of midazolam	Significantly higher doses necessary with the introduction of ECMO; titrate to clinical effect
Sedatives/analgesics: propofol and dexmedetomidine		
Propofol	• LD: 5 µg/kg/min over 5 min • MD: 5–50 µg/kg/min	Significant sequestration within the ECMO circuit	Higher doses may be required; titrate to clinical effect
Dexmedetomidine	• LD: 1 µg/kg over 10 min • MD: 0.2–0.7 µg/kg/h	Losses appear to occur early in the circuit and continue to decline throughout ECMO treatment	Higher doses may be required especially initially; titrate to clinical effect
Antibiotics: vancomycin		

Vancomycin	• LD: 25 mg/kg
	• MD: 15 mg/kg (frequency determined by renal function)
		• Increased Vd and decreased clearance
		• Regimens used in trials:
		  ○ 35 mg/kg loading dose over 4 h followed by a daily infusion adapted to renal function
		  ○ 1 g intravenous loading dose followed by 1 g every 12 h
			Standard dosing recommendations; adjust per therapeutic drug monitoring

Antibiotics: carbapenems		
Imipenem/cilastin	500 mg every 6 h or 1000 mg every 8 h (maximum dose: 4000 mg/d)	• High variability of imipenem trough concentrations • 1 g q 6 h achieved 100% fractional time above the MICs isolated	• Standard dosing recommendations • Higher doses (1 g q 6 h) in patients with resistant organisms and high MICs • Decreased doses in patients with decreased renal function
Meropenem	1–2 g IV q 8 h	Increased Vd; lower clearance	• Standard dosing recommendations • Higher or 2 g q 8 h in patients with resistant organisms and high MICs

(continued on next page)

Table 3
(continued)

Medication	Standard Dosing Recommendations in Critically Ill Patients	Summary of Recommendations in ECMO	Dosing Recommendations for Patients on ECMO Therapy
Antibiotics: piperacillin/tazobactam			
Piperacillin/tazobactam	3.375 IV q 8 h 4-h infusion	No specific dose-adjustment required	• Standard dosing recommendations
Antibiotics: aminoglycosides			
Gentamicin	6 mg/kg IV q 24 h or 1.5 mg/kg IV (frequency determined by renal function)	• Not investigated in adult populations. • Dosing regimens in neonatal population were 25% lower than typical dosing in non-ECMO neonates	Standard dosing approach with monitoring of peak and trough concentration
Amikacin	15 mg/kg IV q 24 h or 7.5 mg/kg IV (frequency determined by renal function)	LD 25 mg/kg dosing based on total body weight (infusion over 30 min) was reported to result in insufficient peak serum concentrations in 25% of patients	Standard dosing approach with therapeutic drug monitoring, with attention to potential for initial low peak
Antibiotics: azithromycin			
Azithromycin	PNA: 500 mg IV daily therapy may be changed to 500 mg PO daily	ECMO does not significantly impact the pharmacokinetics of azithromycin	Standard dosing recommendations
Antibiotics: linezolid			
Linezolid	600 mg IV every 12 h	Pharmacokinetic analyses demonstrated that standard doses were able to achieve adequate AUC/MIC ratios >80 when the organism MIC was ≤1 mg/L; the rate of achieving this parameter decreased when the organism MIC >1 mg/L	Standard dosing recommendations; alternative dosing strategies such as prolonged or continuous infusions have been suggested in critically ill patients in the setting of elevated MICs, although these dosing strategies have not been studied

Antibiotics: tigecycline			
Tigecycline	100 mg IV as a single dose followed by 50 mg IV q 12 h	Standard tigecycline doses are reasonable in patients receiving ECMO	Standard dosing recommendations
Antivirals: oseltamivir			
Oseltamivir	Prophylaxis: 75 mg once daily Treatment: 75 mg twice daily	• Decreased clearance; increased Vd • Limited data suggest that oseltamivir administered orally or by oro/naso gastric tube is well absorbed in critically ill and/or on ECMO	• Standard dosing recommendations • May be administered enteral via oro/naso gastric tube • Decreased doses and therapeutic monitoring in CVVHD patients
Ribavirin	Weight based	• Neonatal data: doses of 20 mg/kg/d IV were associated with low plasma concentrations at steady state	• Standard dosing recommendations • Caution should be exercised due to the lack of data and low plasma concentrations observed in neonates
Antifungals			
Amphotericin B	0.4–1 mg/kg/d depending on indication (formulations not specified in studies)	• ECMO did not contribute to Vd changes • Regimen used in trial: ○ 25 mg IV over 4 h on day 1 followed by 2 1-mg/kg doses separated by 9 h on day 2, and 1 mg/kg/d over 4 h daily starting day 3 (formulations not specified in studies)	Standard dosing recommendations
Caspofungin	70 mg IV on day 1, then 50 mg daily	Not sequestered by the ECMO circuit	Standard dosing recommendations

Voriconazole	IV/PO: 6 mg/kg q 12 h × 2 doses; 4 mg/kg q 12 h	• Significant voriconazole losses in the ECMO circuit (up to 71%)
		• Regimens used in trials:
		  ○ 5.7 mg/kg q 12 h
		  ○ Standard dosing
			Controversial; higher doses of voriconazole required (estimated ~5 mg/kg q 12 h)
			Standard dosing recommendations; due to large interpatient variability, consider 5 mg/kg q 12 h with therapeutic trough monitoring

(continued on next page)

Table 3
(continued)

Medication	Standard Dosing Recommendations in Critically Ill Patients	Summary of Recommendations in ECMO	Dosing Recommendations for Patients on ECMO Therapy
Antituberculosis agents			
Isoniazid, rifampin, ethambutol, and pyrazinamide	Isoniazid: 5 mg/kg/dose (usual dose: 300 mg) once daily Rifampin: 10 mg/kg/d (maximum: 600 mg/d) Ethambutol: 15 mg/kg once daily (maximum dose: 1.5 g) Pyrazinamide: weight based 40–55 kg: 1000 mg 56–75 kg: 1500 mg 76–90 kg: 2000 mg (maximum dose regardless of weight)	Very limited base of evidence on which to make recommendations	• Controversial: 50% increase in doses may be necessary • Use therapeutic drug monitoring to ensure target concentrations

Abbreviations: AUC, area under the curve; CNS, central nervous system; ECMO, extracorporeal membrane oxygenation; IV, intravenous; IVP, IV push; LD, loading dose; MIC, minimum inhibitory concentration; NMDA, N-methyl-D-aspartate; PNA, pneumonia; PO, by mouth; PRN, as needed; q, every; Vd, volume of distribution.

morphine's hydrophilic nature. However, the clearance of morphine decreases up to 50% potentially due to hepatic hypoperfusion.[5,29,30] The accumulation of morphine's active metabolite, especially in renal failure, may lead to prolonged sedation. Furthermore, morphine's histamine release may contribute to bronchospasm and hypotension.[28] Clinicians should be aware of this dynamic accumulation, to allow down titration to clinical effect.[17,29]

Other Opioids

Hydromorphone, a semisynthetic opiate, is an additional option for analgesia and sedation. Although there are no studies investigating its PK in ECMO, hydromorphone is expected to have minimal sequestration within the EMCO circuit due to its hydrophilicity. Unlike morphine, this agent does not have active metabolites and does not cause a histamine release when administered. Although meperidine is a full mu-opioid agonist, it should be avoided due to its potential for drug interactions with serotonergic and dopaminergic agents and metabolite accumulation leading to decreased seizure thresholds.[28]

Ketamine

Adjunctive analgesic medications such as ketamine, an N-methyl-D-aspartate antagonist, are demonstrated to augment opioid analgesia without influencing sympathetic tone.[28,31] In addition to improved wakefulness due to decreased opioid utilization, low-dose ketamine infusions also may offer the advantage of producing amnestic effects. Ketamine has previously demonstrated the ability to decrease opioid or concurrent sedative requirements without altering RASS scores at doses ranging from 50 to 100 mg/h. These high doses may be a result of drug sequestration due to ketamine's lipophilic nature.[32] However, a randomized controlled trial of 20 patients receiving ECMO showed no reduction in opioid or sedative requirements in patients with a low-dose ketamine infusion compared with a control group.[33] Given the paucity and conflicting nature of available data and dosing practices, the optimal use of ketamine in patients receiving ECMO has not yet been defined.

Benzodiazepines

Although opioids alone may provide sufficient analgesia and sedation, some patients may require additional sedation to provide adequate comfort. Benzodiazepines activate gamma-aminobutyric acid receptors leading to anxiolysis, amnesia, and sedation. Midazolam, a benzodiazepine, is frequently used as an infusion given its rapid onset of action, relatively short half-life (2–5 hours), and intermediate duration. Despite being water soluble, midazolam is also highly lipophilic and has been shown to have significant sequestration in the ECMO circuit. Literature suggests that more than 50% of midazolam may be sequestered with most in the first few hours of ECMO initiation. Significantly higher doses of midazolam are necessary with the introduction of ECMO due to this sequestration as well as the increased Vd.[9] Although higher doses may be necessary, accumulation of its active metabolite or liver and renal failure prolong the effect of midazolam, leading to excessive sedation and respiratory depression.[28] This also may contribute to longer recovery times. Lorazepam is less lipophilic than midazolam, leading to a lesser degree of ECMO circuit sequestration.[17] Compared with midazolam, lorazepam has a longer half-life of 10 to 20 hours and does not have any active metabolites. However, caution is warranted, especially in using high doses and for prolonged periods due to the polyethylene glycol excipient that can cause potential renal toxicity.

Propofol and Dexmedetomidine

Nonbenzodiazepine sedatives also may be used in conjunction with opioids to provide additional sedation. Propofol, a lipophilic and highly protein-bound agent, has been found to have significant sequestration within the ECMO circuit.[34] This makes propofol possibility a less desirable agent for sedative therapy for patients receiving ECMO.[28] Dexmedetomidine, an alpha 2-adrenergic agonist, has analgesic, anxiolytic, and sedative properties. Patients sedated with dexmedetomidine are easily aroused. Compared with benzodiazepines, dexmedetomidine is associated with a reduced incidence of delirium, respiratory depression, and impact on sympathetic tone.[27,35] If the patient requires deep sedation due to neuromuscular blockade, dexmedetomidine is not appropriate in monotherapy. Dexmedetomidine sequestration appears to occur early in the circuit and continues to decline throughout ECMO treatment. Despite these losses, the clearance of dexmedetomidine between old and new circuits has not been found to be statistically significant. Thus, dexmedetomidine may experience medication losses in ECMO circuits, either through sequestration or clearance. Dexmedetomidine therapy in patients receiving ECMO requires monitoring and appropriate dose adjustments to ensure adequate serum concentrations.[36]

The approach to analgesia and sedation for patients receiving ECMO should be patient specific. Choice of drug depends on level of sedation required due to the presence of neuromuscular blocking agents or instrumentation, patient characteristics such as previous drug exposure or tolerance, expected duration of therapy, and allergies. Institutional formulary restrictions, drug cost, shortages, and local guidelines also help to guide therapy.

NEUROMUSCULAR BLOCKADE

Neuromuscular blocking agents (NMBAs) may be used in patients receiving ECMO in conjunction with sedatives to provide pharmacologic skeletal muscle paralysis. These agents should be reserved for select situations in which paralysis is necessary to improve patient-ventilator synchrony, enhance alveoli recruitment and oxygenation, and reduce overall oxygen demand.[37,38] Clinical practice patterns of pharmacologic paralysis in patients receiving ECMO is variable.[24,25] Currently, there are no PK data available to tailor NMBA dosing for patients receiving ECMO. Standard dosing and appropriate titration are recommended. Peripheral nerve stimulation testing, such as train of 4 monitoring is vital for paralytic assessment and NMBA titration.[39] Patients receiving neuromuscular blockade must be also monitored for symptoms of ICU-acquired weakness, myopathy, and polyneuropathy.[40]

ANTICOAGULATION

As blood is exposed to nonbiological surfaces and high shear stress, platelet activation and the coagulation cascade is triggered, putting patients at risk for clotting during ECMO.[41–43] Additional factors provoking hypercoagulability during ECMO therapy include cannulation-induced endothelial injury and blood flow disturbances.[44] Even in settings of a variety of different pumps, membrane oxygenators, heat exchangers, and priming volumes, the overall impact on hemostasis is largely consistent.[41,45] Methods such as coating nonendothelial surfaces with anticoagulants and systemic anticoagulation have been investigated to minimize the risk of thrombosis. Unfractionated heparin (UFH) is a standard and widely used anticoagulant. There is no standard dose of heparin currently recommended. Although sites may have institution-specific protocols for infusing UFH during ECMO, one method is to administer a heparin bolus of

50–70 units/kg at the time of vascular cannula insertion followed by a continuous infusion initiated at 18 units/kg per hour titrated to a goal activated partial thromboplastin time (aPTT) of 50 to 60 seconds.[41] Therapeutic targets vary according to institution. An international survey investigating current practices of anticoagulation in patients receiving ECMO has found that activated clotting time (ACT), antithrombin III, anti-factor Xa, and thromboelastography may be alternatives for anticoagulation monitoring.[46] None of these are readily available at most institutions and their use has not been established to achieve better clinical outcomes than the use of PTT monitoring. Optimal targets for anticoagulation in patients receiving ECMO remain unclear due to the delicate balance between thrombotic and hemorrhagic complications.[47] Large systematic reviews have noted the rate of thrombosis in patients receiving VV ECMO to be 53%. Conversely, rates of gastrointestinal or intracranial hemorrhage in patients receiving VV ECMO have been reported to be approximately 16%.[41,47] Thrombotic and hemorrhagic rates have not yet been quantified in patients receiving VA ECMO. In attempts to minimize bleeding complications, there have been reports of patients with heparin-coated ECMO circuits who have successfully omitted additional systemic anticoagulation without increasing thrombotic risk.[48,49] Furthermore, heparin-free ECMO may be a consideration in select patients with severe trauma or extensive bleeding risks.[50,51] The use of UFH as well as specific titration endpoints should be tailored to each patient's individualized thrombotic and hemorrhagic risk factors.

Although heparin is a suitable anticoagulant for most patients, 10% to 15% of patients receiving ECMO have reported heparin-induced thrombocytopenia (HIT).[38] Heparin needs to be discontinued in this group of patients.[52] Direct thrombin inhibitors, such as argatroban and bivalirudin are alternative agents for patients receiving ECMO who have HIT.[38,53–57] The necessity of an initial argatroban bolus is controversial. Argatroban may be bolused with a range of 10 to 30 μg. Case reports have documented patients receiving ECMO to initiate standard doses of argatroban at 2 μg/kg per minute and subsequently titrate to aPTT levels 1.5 to 3.0 times baseline without significant bleeding concerns.[23] However, other reports note that typical argatroban infusion rates of 2 μg/kg per minute have been associated with excessive anticoagulation and severe bleeding in patients receiving ECMO. Comparatively, 10-fold lower dosages of 0.2 μg/kg per minute have been demonstrated to achieve appropriate levels of anticoagulation, defined as an aPTT range of 50 to 60 seconds.[58,59] An additional case report notes that a starting dose of argatroban between 0.1 and 0.2 μg/kg per minute resulted in adequate anticoagulation without any thrombotic or hemorrhagic complications in a patient with high bleeding risk as defined by a dosing weight greater than 90 kg, bilirubin greater than 51.3 mmol/L, and platelet count less than 70×10^9/L.[60] Due to the lack of a consensus dosing method, it may be recommended to initiate argatroban at lower doses, especially in patients at high risk of bleeding. Critically ill patients who are not receiving ECMO also often have a variable dose response to argatroban, leading some clinicians to use regimens of 1.0 or 0.5 μg/kg per minute as initial therapy. Bivalirudin is not preferred for all patients because of its high cost and lack of an antidote. Previous studies have used bivalirudin with or without a bolus loading dose followed by an infusion ranging from 0.1 to 0.2 mg/kg per hour to 0.5 mg/kg per hour. Similar to heparin, there is no consensus for bivalirudin monitoring parameters. Reported monitoring strategies during bivalirudin therapy have ranged from aPTT 45 to 60 seconds to 42 to 88 seconds, ACT 180 to 200 seconds to 200 to 220 seconds, and thromboelastography.[61]

The use of additional antithrombotic agents to minimize platelet activation and deposition in patients receiving ECMO should be evaluated on a case to case basis.[62] Aspirin, an irreversible cyclooxygenase (COX) inhibitor, is often recommended for the prevention of primary or secondary cardiovascular events. In patients receiving ECMO, aspirin also may be beneficial to reduce platelet binding to the circuit.[63] Adjunctive aspirin use in a single prospective cohort study with patients receiving ECMO was not found to increase bleeding or transfusion requirements.[64] Indication for aspirin should be individualized in patients with coagulation disorders or moderate to severe traumatic brain injury. Clopidogrel, an irreversible inhibitor of the $P2Y_{12}$ component of ADP receptors on platelets, has been evaluated in a small subset of patients with acute coronary syndrome receiving ECMO therapy. Although clopidogrel therapy may be associated with increased transfusion requirements, it has not been associated with a significant bleeding risk.[65,66] Generally, dual antiplatelet therapy in patients with recent coronary stent implantation should not be withheld.[63,67,68] Glycoprotein IIb/IIIa inhibitors also may be used in patients receiving VA ECMO with recent percutaneous coronary interventions. One retrospective observational study found that patients receiving ECMO on glycoprotein IIb/IIIa inhibitors required an increased number of transfusions.[65] The benefit and risk of additional antithrombotic agents should be evaluated on a case-by-case basis.

ANTIBIOTICS

Antimicrobial regimens that optimize drug exposure relative to therapeutic concentrations maximize antimicrobial efficacy and decrease toxicity. More than other drug classes, antibiotic concentration is an effective biomarker linked to therapeutic success when extrapolating drug dosing between populations. This is the case in ECMO, in which there is a lack of comparative efficacy data to guide therapeutics. Although several antibiotics have been analyzed, few trials have been conducted in the adult ECMO population. Among the available studies in adult patients receiving ECMO, results have demonstrated significant interpatient variability.[10,14,19,69]

Vancomycin

Vancomycin, a glycopeptide antimicrobial, is a widely used broad-spectrum agent with activity against Staphylococcus, Streptococcus, and Enterococcus species. Vancomycin PK may be estimated by a ratio of the area under the concentration-time curve (AUC) to the minimum inhibitory concentration (MIC).[70] A consensus review from the American Society of Health-System Pharmacists, the Infectious Diseases Society of America, and the Society of Infectious Diseases Pharmacists has established a vancomycin PK/PD parameter of an AUC/MIC ratio greater than 400 for serious infections. It is estimated that targeting vancomycin trough levels of 15 to 20 mg/L should achieve this AUC for organisms with relatively low MICs (MIC ≤1 mg/L). Suggested vancomycin dosing to achieve these trough levels and ultimately AUC/MIC ratios includes a loading dose of 25 to 30 mg/kg based on actual body weight followed by a maintenance dose of 15 to 20 mg/kg every 8 to 12 hours in patients with normal renal function. Individual PK adjustments should be made based on therapeutic drug monitoring.[71] Although the PK parameters of vancomycin have been heavily studied, most trials in patients receiving ECMO have investigated only pediatric and neonatal populations. Recent studies with mixed populations, including neonates, children, and adults, suggest an increased Vd and decreased clearance of vancomycin during ECMO therapy.[20] Despite these changes in PK parameters, adult population models derived from smaller trials have found that no special dosing adjustments are required in patients receiving ECMO. Pharmacometric modeling has demonstrated that standard dosing regimens may be adequate in achieving therapeutic trough concentrations, especially in obese patients on ECMO therapy.[72] Nevertheless, standard vancomycin dosing regimens vary per institution. Some centers have investigated a 35-mg/kg loading dose over 4 hours followed by a daily infusion adapted to creatinine clearance and renal function, whereas others have used an initial 1-g IV dose followed by 1 g every 12 hours.[73,74] The presence of renal dysfunction and interventions such as continuous RRT or hemodialysis further complicate vancomycin dosing. Given the mixed data, interpatient variability, and differences among ECMO circuits, therapeutic drug monitoring is essential to ensure optimal vancomycin levels.[75]

Carbapenems

Carbapenems are members of the beta-lactam class of antibiotics and are typically reserved for multidrug-resistant bacteria. Beta-lactams, including carbapenems, exert time-dependent killing. These time-dependent antibiotics rely on the amount of time that the antibiotic serum concentration remains above the organism's MIC.[76] Carbapenems undergo many PK alterations during ECMO, including Vd changes and significant sequestration within the EMCO circuit.[77] Limited studies are available to describe changes in carbapenem PK parameters in patients receiving ECMO. The high variability of imipenem trough concentrations has been described in a case report of lung transplant patients on VV ECMO who received imipenem 1 g every 6 hours. These reports note that using the dosing regimen of 1 g every 6 hours achieved 100% fractional time above the MICs isolated in the patients studied. Patients with resistant organisms and high MICs may require higher doses, and patients with decreased renal function may need dose reductions.[78] The PK of meropenem in patients receiving ECMO also has been investigated. Meropenem use in patients receiving ECMO has been associated with an increased Vd, yet a lower clearance. Meropenem clearance has been found to correlate with creatinine clearance and the presence of RRT. Ultimately, standard dosing regimens with 1 g every 8 hours are expected to yield routine target concentrations. However, increased doses may be necessary when targeting less susceptible microorganisms.[79] To further address dosing regimens with resistant organisms, direct comparisons have been drawn between a VV ECMO patient with *Enterobacter* septicemia receiving meropenem 1 g every 8 hours and a VA ECMO patient with *Pseudomonas aeruginosa* pneumonia (MIC 2 mg/L) and multiorgan failure receiving a high-dose meropenem infusion of 6.5 g every 24 hours. Similar to previous findings, the standard 1 g every 8 hours regimen was sufficient for organisms with lower MICs; however, increased dosages, such as the high-dose infusion, were necessary to achieve adequate concentrations for resistant organisms.[12]

Piperacillin/Tazobactam

Many critically ill patients may require treatment with broad-spectrum β-lactams and, similarly to carbapenems, the PK parameters of β-lactams during EMCO are not well investigated. Piperacillin/tazobactam is a β-lactam/β-lactamase inhibitor antibiotic with time-dependent activity commonly used for empiric broad-spectrum therapy. Recent investigations using therapeutic drug monitoring of piperacillin/tazobactam concentrations in patients on ECMO therapy demonstrate no significant differences in PK parameters between ECMO and patients not receiving ECMO. Although limited, these data suggest that dose adjustments are not required with piperacillin/tazobactam during ECMO therapy.[80]

Aminoglycosides

Aminoglycosides, including gentamicin, tobramycin, and amikacin, are broad-spectrum antibiotics with concentration-dependent bactericidal activity. Ensuring adequate peak and trough levels are essential to optimize antimicrobial killing while minimizing toxicity.

Gentamicin PK data derived from neonatal ECMO populations suggest a significantly increased Vd and half-life, as well as a decreased clearance. These PK variations may be a result of gentamicin's hydrophilic profile as well as the decreased renal perfusion seen in neonates, especially during nonpulsatile ECMO therapy. Recommended dosing regimens in this neonatal population are typically 25% lower than typical dosing in non-ECMO neonates.[5,9,10,14,17] Although tobramycin has not been separately investigated, because of its comparable PK profile to gentamicin, similar dosing recommendations may be applied. PK parameters and dosage recommendations for gentamicin and tobramycin have not been investigated in adult populations. Given the differences in total body water content and renal clearance between neonates and adults, findings in the neonatal population cannot be extrapolated to adults. Because of the lack of data in adult populations, standard dosing regimens for both gentamicin and tobramycin should be used. Given the lack of data in adult patients, close therapeutic monitoring of gentamicin peak and trough levels should be performed.

In contrast to gentamicin, amikacin has been investigated in adult populations. In a single study, ECMO has not been found to significantly impact amikacin peak and trough levels. These data stem from adult patients on VA or VV ECMO receiving an amikacin 25 mg/kg loading dose based on total body weight as an infusion over 30 minutes. It is important to note that this loading dose of 25 mg/kg was reported to result in insufficient peak serum concentrations in 25% of patients. Similar to gentamicin, it can be recommended to continue standard amikacin dosing regimens in patients receiving ECMO with therapeutic drug monitoring.[81,82]

Azithromycin

Azithromycin, a macrolide antibiotic with a long half-life, has been briefly investigated among adult patients receiving VV ECMO with preserved renal function. Patients received standard doses of 500 mg IV every 24 hours. PK parameters, including maximum and minimum concentrations as well as the AUC, were similar to patients not receiving ECMO. Furthermore, the assessment of blood samples collected at steady state revealed a similar clearance but a decreased Vd as compared with healthy volunteers. Collectively, these results suggest that ECMO does not significantly impact the PK of azithromycin.[83]

Linezolid

Linezolid is a protein synthesis inhibitor that is typically reserved for resistant gram-positive infections, such as vancomycin-resistant *Enterococcus* and specific cases of methicillin-resistant *Staphylococcus aureus* (MRSA). Because of its high pulmonary penetration, linezolid is a reasonable therapeutic option for pneumonia caused by these resistant organisms. Only one report has investigated linezolid plasma concentrations in patients on ECMO. This report investigated linezolid PK parameters in 3 adult patients being treated for MRSA pneumonia. *S aureus* MICs ranged from 1 mg/L to 4 mg/L and each patient received standard doses of linezolid 600 mg IV every 12 hours. Pharmacokinetic analyses demonstrated that standard doses were able to achieve adequate AUC/MIC ratios greater than 80 only when the MIC was ≤1 mg/L.[84] Although limited data are available, it is recommended to continue standard dosing when the MIC is ≤1 mg/L. In instances in which the MIC is >1 mg/L, previous studies suggest the use of prolonged or continuous infusions as well as increased dosages of linezolid.

Tigecycline

Tigecycline, a glycylcycline antibiotic typically reserved for resistant infections, has a very large Vd, and is eliminated primarily unchanged in feces and urine. To date, there is only 1 case report investigating tigecycline PK in patients receiving ECMO. Tigecycline treatment has been described in an adult patient receiving VV ECMO with a persistent *Staphylococcus epidermidis* pulmonary infection in the setting of vancomycin resistance. This specific patient received standard tigecycline doses of 50 mg IV twice daily. Through measurements of plasma and tracheal aspirate concentrations, it was determined that ECMO does not have an impact on tigecycline PK.[85] The available data suggest standard tigecycline doses may be used in patients receiving ECMO.

Oseltamivir

Oseltamivir, an antiviral medication, is indicated for the treatment and prophylaxis of influenza. The standard dose of oseltamivir for the treatment of influenza is 75 mg administered nasogastrically or nasoenterically every 12 hours. Similar to the absorption of parenteral medications through the ECMO circuit, the absorption of enteral medications is also variable. Limited data suggest oseltamivir is adequately absorbed when enterally administered during ECMO.[86,87] Pharmacokinetic parameters of oseltamivir administered nasogastrically or nasoenterically in patients receiving ECMO include decreased clearance and increased Vd compared with healthy adult patients. Although specific dosage adjustments for ECMO are not necessary, oseltamivir still should be adjusted for renal impairment.[88] The effects of continuous venovenous hemodialysis (CVVHD) in addition to ECMO therapy have also been investigated. PK of oseltamivir and oseltamivir carboxylate in patients concurrently on CVVHD and ECMO revealed no substantial differences between pre-ECMO and post-ECMO oxygenator plasma concentrations. Although ECMO may not extensively contribute to changes in oseltamivir PK, CVVHD significantly affects its clearance.[89] Standard doses of oseltamivir in patients on CVVHD have been associated with drug accumulation. Thus, decreased oseltamivir doses are recommended in patients with renal failure and in patients requiring CVVHD. No specific dosage adjustments are necessary during ECMO therapy.[88,90]

Ribavirin

Ribavirin, an antiviral medication, has been used for the treatment of disseminated adenovirus in neonates requiring hemofiltration. Doses of 20 mg/kg per day IV have demonstrated low plasma concentrations at steady state despite negative viral cultures 48 hours after ribavirin initiation.[91] Additional studies in the adult population have yet to be conducted. Standard dosing recommendations may be used in adult patients receiving ECMO; caution should be exercised because of the lack of data and low plasma concentrations observed in neonates.

ANTIFUNGALS
Amphotericin B

Amphotericin B is a polyene antifungal agent that binds to ergosterol in the fungal cell wall leading to alterations in cell membrane permeability. Only 1 case report of IV amphotericin B use in one 15-year-old patient on VA ECMO with respiratory failure secondary to *Blastomyces dermatitidis* pneumonia has been reported. The specific formulation of IV amphotericin B was not specified. The patient received 25 mg IV over 4 hours on the first day of therapy followed by two 100-mg (1 mg/kg) doses separated by 9 hours on day 2, and 100 mg over 4 hours daily (1 mg/kg per day) starting on day 3. Analysis of the patient's amphotericin B peak and trough levels indicate that ECMO did not contribute to Vd changes affecting amphotericin B therapy. Based on this limited data set, no specific dosing adjustments need to be made in patients receiving ECMO.[92,93]

Echinocandins/Azoles

Fungal infections in ICUs have risen significantly in the past several decades. Broad-spectrum antifungal agents, such as caspofungin and voriconazole, may be used as empiric therapy for specific at-risk ICU patient populations. Ex vivo studies in blood-primed ECMO circuits have demonstrated significant voriconazole losses up to 71%.[11] Because of this anticipated voriconazole sequestration, voriconazole doses in an in vivo study were increased from 280 mg (4 mg/kg) twice daily to 400 mg (6 mg/kg) twice daily. Drug concentration obtained 2 days after this dose increase reflected supratherapeutic levels with troughs greater than 10 mg/mL and peaks of approximately 15 mg/mL. The analysis of caspofungin peaks and troughs in these patients suggest that caspofungin is not sequestered by the ECMO circuit.[94] Comparatively, an additional case report notes a patient to receive standard doses of voriconazole (6 mg/kg twice daily on day 1 followed by 4 mg/kg twice daily) and caspofungin (70 mg on day 1 followed by 50 mg/d). Blood concentrations collected for both voriconazole and caspofungin revealed undetectable circulating levels.[93] It is difficult to draw a conclusion based on these 2 reports. Voriconazole has demonstrated significant interpatient variability even among nonpatients receiving ECMO.[95] Additional studies elucidating the effect of voriconazole PK in patients receiving ECMO are necessary. Therapeutic drug monitoring should be conducted in all patients receiving ECMO on voriconazole therapy to ensure efficacy and to minimize toxicity. Data suggest that standard-dosed caspofungin may be adequate in patients receiving ECMO. In light of limited data, dosing recommendations are provisional for these agents.

Antituberculosis Agents

A case report of 1 adult patient on VV ECMO documents subtherapeutic levels of isoniazid, rifampin, ethambutol, and pyrazinamide despite standard dosing regimens. To achieve target plasma concentrations, the patient required conversion from oral to IV administration routes and doses of 23 mg/kg per day of rifampin (compared with the standard dose of 10 mg/kg per day). Double the standard doses of pyrazinamide and ethambutol were also necessary.[62] The PK parameters of ethambutol and rifampin also have been investigated in patients on ECMO and extended daily dialysis. Contrary to the case report previously described, results from the PK analysis conclude that the ECMO membrane did not have an effect on the removal of either medication. However, extended daily dialysis removed a considerable amount of both medications from circulating volume. Ethambutol doses between 1000 and 2000 mg/d are suggested for patients on RRT to achieve target peak levels.[96] These conflicting data support the use of therapeutic drug monitoring in patients receiving ECMO to ensure target concentrations.

SUMMARY

PK changes resulting from ECMO and their clinical impact are not yet fully characterized for most of the drugs used in critically ill patients. Given the limited patient population, the database of PK studies in patients receiving ECMO is largely reliant on in vitro data or case studies. Although limited, available data can assist health care providers in tailoring dosing regimens for adult patients receiving ECMO. Whenever possible, therapeutic drug monitoring should be conducted to ensure efficacy while minimizing toxicity.

REFERENCES

1. Boucher BA, Wood GC, Swanson JM. Pharmacokinetic changes in critical illness. Crit Care Clin 2006;22(2):255–71.
2. Vilay AM, Churchwell MD, Mueller BA. Clinical review: drug metabolism and non-renal clearance in acute kidney injury. Crit Care 2008;12(6):235.
3. Schmith VD, Foss JF. Inflammation: planning for a source of pharmacokinetic/pharmacodynamic variability in translational studies. Clin Pharmacol Ther 2010; 87(4):488–91.
4. Smith BS, Yogaratnam D, Levasseur-Franklin KE, et al. Introduction to drug pharmacokinetics in the critically ill patient. Chest 2012;141(5):1327–36.
5. Mousavi S, Levcovich B, Mojtahedzadeh M. A systematic review on pharmacokinetic changes in critically ill patients: role of extracorporeal membrane oxygenation. Daru 2011;19(5):312–21. Available at: http://daru.tums.ac.ir/index.php/daru/article/view/409.
6. Hadidi E, Mojtahedzadeh M, Rouini MR, et al. The evaluation of the possible effect of positive end expiratory pressure (PEEP) on pharmacokinetics of phenytoin in patients with acute brain injury under mechanical ventilation. DARU J Pharm Sci 2005;13(2):74–81.
7. Anderson HL, Coran AG, Drongowski RA, et al. Extracellular fluid and total body water changes in neonates undergoing extracorporeal membrane oxygenation. J Pediatr Surg 1992;27(8):1003–8.
8. Perkins MW, Dasta JF, Dehaven B. Physiologic implications of mechanical ventilation on pharmacokinetics. DICP 1989;23(4):316–23. Available at: http://journals.sagepub.com/doi/abs/10.1177/106002808902300408.
9. Shekar K, Roberts JA, Welch S, et al. ASAP ECMO: antibiotic, sedative and analgesic pharmacokinetics during extracorporeal membrane oxygenation: a multicentre study to optimise drug therapy during ECMO. BMC Anesthesiol 2012; 12:29.
10. Buck ML. Pharmacokinetic changes during extracorporeal membrane oxygenation: implications for drug therapy of neonates. Clin Pharmacokinet 2003;42(5): 403–17.
11. Mehta NM, Halwick DR, Dodson BL, et al. Potential drug sequestration during extracorporeal membrane oxygenation: results from an ex vivo experiment. Intensive Care Med 2007;33(6):1018–24.
12. Shekar K, Roberts JA, Ghassabian S, et al. Altered antibiotic pharmacokinetics during extracorporeal membrane oxygenation: cause for concern? J Antimicrob Chemother 2013;68(3):726–7.
13. Rosen DA, Rosen KR, Silvasi DL. In vitro variability in fentanyl absorption by different membrane oxygenators. J Cardiothorac Anesth 1990;4(3):332–5.

14. Dagan O, Klein J, Gruenwald C, et al. Preliminary studies of the effects of extra-corporeal membrane oxygenator on the disposition of common pediatric drugs. Ther Drug Monit 1993;15(4):263–6.

15. Wildschut ED, Ahsman MJ, Allegaert K, et al. Determinants of drug absorption in different ECMO circuits. Intensive Care Med 2010;36(12):2109–16. Available at: http://www.ncbi.nlm.nih.gov/pmc/articles/PMC2981740/.

16. Preston TJ, Hodge AB, Riley JB, et al. In vitro drug adsorption and plasma free hemoglobin levels associated with hollow fiber oxygenators in the extracorporeal life support (ECLS) circuit. J Extra Corpor Technol 2007;39(4):234–7. Available at: http://www.ncbi.nlm.nih.gov/pmc/articles/PMC4680688/.

17. Bhatt-Meht V, Annich G. Sedative clearance during extracorporeal membrane oxygenation. Perfusion 2005;20(6):309–15.

18. Shekar K, Roberts JA, Mcdonald CI, et al. Protein-bound drugs are prone to sequestration in the extracorporeal membrane oxygenation circuit: results from an ex vivo study. Crit Care 2015;19(1):164.

19. Shekar K, Fraser JF, Smith MT, et al. Pharmacokinetic changes in patients receiving extracorporeal membrane oxygenation. J Crit Care 2012;27(6): 741.e9-18.

20. Mulla H, Lawson G, von Anrep C, et al. In vitro evaluation of sedative drug losses during extracorporeal membrane oxygenation. Perfusion 2000;15(1):21–6. Available at: http://journals.sagepub.com/doi/abs/10.1177/026765910001500104.

21. Paden ML, Conrad SA, Rycus PT, et al, ELSO Registry. Extracorporeal life support organization registry report 2012. ASAIO J 2013;59(3):202–10.

22. Roos JF, Bulitta J, Lipman J, et al. Pharmacokinetic-pharmacodynamic rationale for cefepime dosing regimens in intensive care units. J Antimicrob Chemother 2006;58(5):987–93.

23. Johnston N, Wait M, Huber L. Argatroban in adult extracorporeal membrane oxygenation. J Extra Corpor Technol 2002;34(4):281–4.

24. Buscher H, Vaidiyanathan SF, Al-Soufi SF, et al. Sedation practice in veno-venous extracorporeal membrane oxygenation: an international survey. ASAIO J 2013; 59(6):636–41.

25. DeGrado JR, Hohlfelder B, Ritchie BM, et al. Evaluation of sedatives, analgesics, and neuromuscular blocking agents in adults receiving extracorporeal membrane oxygenation. J Crit Care 2017;37:1–6.

26. Erstad BL, Puntillo K, Gilbert HC, et al. Pain management principles in the critically ill. Chest 2009;135(4):1075–86.

27. Barr J, Fraser GL, Puntillo KF, et al. Clinical practice guidelines for the management of pain, agitation, and delirium in adult patients in the intensive care unit. Crit Care Med 2013;41(1):263–306.

28. Satyapriya SV, Lyaker ML, Rozycki AJ, et al. Sedation, analgesia delirium in the ECMO patient. In: Firstenberg MS, editor. Extracorporeal membrane oxygenation—advances in therapy. Rijeka (Croatia): InTech; 2016. p. 287–304.

29. Dagan O, Klein JF, Bohn DF, et al. Effects of extracorporeal membrane oxygenation on morphine pharmacokinetics in infants. Crit Care Med 1994;22(7): 1099–101.

30. Peters JWB, Anderson BJ, Simons SHP, et al. Morphine pharmacokinetics during venoarterial extracorporeal membrane oxygenation in neonates. Intensive Care Med 2005;31(2):257–63.

31. Subramaniam K, Subramaniam B, Steinbrook RA. Ketamine as adjuvant analgesic to opioids: a quantitative and qualitative systematic review. Anesth Analg 2004;99(2):482–95. Table of contents.

32. Tellor B, Shin N, Graetz TJ, et al. Ketamine infusion for patients receiving extracorporeal membrane oxygenation support: a case series [version 1; referees: 2 approved]. F1000Res 2015;4:16. Available at: http://f1000r.es/4yj.

33. Dzierba AL, Brodie D, Bacchetta M, et al. Ketamine use in sedation management in patients receiving extracorporeal membrane oxygenation. Intensive Care Med 2016;42(11):1822–3.

34. Hynynen M, Hammaren E, Rosenberg PH. Propofol sequestration within the extracorporeal circuit. Can J Anaesth 1994;41(7):583.

35. Riker RR, Shehabi Y, Bokesch PM, et al. Dexmedetomidine vs midazolam for sedation of critically ill patients: a randomized trial. JAMA 2009;301(5):489–99.

36. Wagner D, Pasko D, Phillips K, et al. In vitro clearance of dexmedetomidine in extracorporeal membrane oxygenation. Perfusion 2013;28(1):40–6. Available at: http://journals.sagepub.com/doi/abs/10.1177/0267659112456894.

37. Hraiech S, Dizier S, Papazian L. The use of paralytics in patients with acute respiratory distress syndrome. Clin Chest Med 2014;35(4):753–63.

38. Tulman DB, Stawicki SPA, Whitson BA, et al. Veno-venous ECMO: a synopsis of nine key potential challenges, considerations, and controversies. BMC Anesthesiol 2014;14:65. Available at: http://www.ncbi.nlm.nih.gov/pmc/articles/PMC4126084/.

39. Greenberg SB, Vender J. The use of neuromuscular blocking agents in the ICU: where are we now? Crit Care Med 2013;41(5):1332–44.

40. Latronico N, Guarneri B. Critical illness myopathy and neuropathy. Minerva Anestesiol 2008;74(6):319–23.

41. Protti A, L'Acqua C, Panigada M. The delicate balance between pro- (risk of thrombosis) and anti- (risk of bleeding) coagulation during extracorporeal membrane oxygenation. Ann Transl Med 2016;4(7):139. Available at: http://www.ncbi.nlm.nih.gov/pmc/articles/PMC4842390/.

42. Oliver WC. Anticoagulation and coagulation management for ECMO. Semin Cardiothorac Vasc Anesth 2009;13(3):154–75. Available at: http://journals.sagepub.com/doi/abs/10.1177/1089253209347384.

43. Muntean W. Coagulation and anticoagulation in extracorporeal membrane oxygenation. Artif Organs 1999;23(11):979–83.

44. Trudzinski FC, Minko P, Rapp D, et al. Runtime and aPTT predict venous thrombosis and thromboembolism in patients on extracorporeal membrane oxygenation: a retrospective analysis. Ann Intensive Care 2016;6(1):66.

45. Malfertheiner MV, Philipp A, Lubnow M, et al. Hemostatic changes during extracorporeal membrane oxygenation: a prospective randomized clinical trial comparing three different extracorporeal membrane oxygenation systems. Crit Care Med 2016;44(4):747–54.

46. Bembea MM, Annich G, Rycus P, et al. Variability in anticoagulation management of patients on extracorporeal membrane oxygenation: an international survey. Pediatr Crit Care Med 2013;14(2):e77–84. Available at: http://www.ncbi.nlm.nih.gov/pmc/articles/PMC3567253/.

47. Sklar MC, Sy E, Lequier L, et al. Anticoagulation practices during venovenous extracorporeal membrane oxygenation for respiratory failure. A systematic review. Ann Am Thorac Soc 2016;13(12):2242–50.

48. Lamarche Y, Chow B, Bedard A, et al. Thromboembolic events in patients on extracorporeal membrane oxygenation without anticoagulation. Innovations (Phila) 2010;5(6):424–9.

49. Krueger K, Schmutz A, Zieger B, et al. Venovenous extracorporeal membrane oxygenation with prophylactic subcutaneous anticoagulation only: an observational study in more than 60 patients. Artif Organs 2017;41(2):186–92.

50. Wen PH, Chan WH, Chen YC, et al. Non-heparinized ECMO serves a rescue method in a multitrauma patient combining pulmonary contusion and nonoperative internal bleeding: a case report and literature review. World J Emerg Surg 2015;10:15.

51. Arlt M, Philipp A, Voelkel S, et al. Extracorporeal membrane oxygenation in severe trauma patients with bleeding shock. Resuscitation 2010;81(7):804–9.

52. Chung YS, Cho DY, Sohn DS, et al. Is stopping heparin safe in patients on extracorporeal membrane oxygenation treatment? ASAIO J 2017;63(1):32–6.

53. Koster A, Weng Y, Bottcher W, et al. Successful use of bivalirudin as anticoagulant for ECMO in a patient with acute HIT. Ann Thorac Surg 2007;83(5):1865–7.

54. Ranucci M, Ballotta A, Kandil H, et al. Bivalirudin-based versus conventional heparin anticoagulation for postcardiotomy extracorporeal membrane oxygenation. Crit Care 2011;15(6):R275. Available at: http://www.ncbi.nlm.nih.gov/pmc/articles/PMC3388709/.

55. Pieri M, Agracheva N, Bonaveglio E, et al. Bivalirudin versus heparin as an anticoagulant during extracorporeal membrane oxygenation: a case-control study. J Cardiothorac Vasc Anesth 2013;27(1):30–4.

56. Young G, Yonekawa KE, Nakagawa P, et al. Argatroban as an alternative to heparin in extracorporeal membrane oxygenation circuits. Perfusion 2004;19(5):283–8.

57. Kawada T, Kitagawa H, Hoson M, et al. Clinical application of argatroban as an alternative anticoagulant for extracorporeal circulation. Hematol Oncol Clin North Am 2000;14(2):445–57.

58. Beiderlinden M, Treschan T, Görlinger K, et al. Argatroban in extracorporeal membrane oxygenation. Artif Organs 2007;31(6):461–5.

59. Potter KE, Raj A, Sullivan JE. Argatroban for anticoagulation in pediatric patients with heparin-induced thrombocytopenia requiring extracorporeal life support. J Pediatr Hematol Oncol 2007;29(4):265–8.

60. Phillips MR, Khoury AI, Ashton RF, et al. The dosing and monitoring of argatroban for heparin-induced thrombocytopenia during extracorporeal membrane oxygenation: a word of caution. Anaesth Intensive Care 2014;42(1):97–8.

61. Sanfilippo F, Asmussen S, Maybauer DM, et al. Bivalirudin for alternative anticoagulation in extracorporeal membrane oxygenation: a systematic review. J Intensive Care Med 2017;32(5):312–9.

62. Kim HS, Lee ES, Cho YJ. Insufficient serum levels of antituberculosis agents during venovenous extracorporeal membrane oxygenation therapy for acute respiratory distress syndrome in a patient with miliary tuberculosis. ASAIO J 2014;60(4):484–6.

63. Glauber M, Szefner J, Senni M, et al. Reduction of haemorrhagic complications during mechanically assisted circulation with the use of a multi-system anticoagulation protocol. Int J Artif Organs 1995;18(10):649–55.

64. Bein T, Zimmermann M, Philipp A, et al. Addition of acetylsalicylic acid to heparin for anticoagulation management during pumpless extracorporeal lung assist. ASAIO J 2011;57(3):164–8.

65. Esper SA, Bermudez C, Dueweke EJ, et al. Extracorporeal membrane oxygenation support in acute coronary syndromes complicated by cardiogenic shock. Catheter Cardiovasc Interv 2015;86(Suppl 1):S45–50.

66. Barthelemy O, Silvain J, Brieger D, et al. Bleeding complications in primary percutaneous coronary intervention of ST-elevation myocardial infarction in a radial center. Catheter Cardiovasc Interv 2012;79(1):104–12.

67. Szefner J. Control and treatment of hemostasis in cardiovascular surgery. the experience of La Pitié Hospital with patients on total artificial heart. Int J Artif Organs 1995;18(10):633–48.

68. Staudacher DL, Biever PM, Benk C, et al. Dual antiplatelet therapy (DAPT) versus no antiplatelet therapy and incidence of major bleeding in patients on venoarterial extracorporeal membrane oxygenation. PLoS One 2016;11(7):e0159973.

69. Sherwin J, Heath T, Watt K. Pharmacokinetics and dosing of anti-infective drugs in patients on extracorporeal membrane oxygenation: a review of the current literature. Clin Ther 2016;38(9):1976–94.

70. Brown DL, Lalla CD, Masselink AJ. AUC versus peak-trough dosing of vancomycin: applying new pharmacokinetic paradigms to an old drug. Ther Drug Monit 2013;35(4):443–9.

71. Rybak MJ, Lomaestro BM, Rotschafer JC, et al. Vancomycin therapeutic guidelines: a summary of consensus recommendations from the Infectious Diseases Society of America, the American Society of Health-System Pharmacists, and the Society of Infectious Diseases Pharmacists. Clin Infect Dis 2009;49(3):325–7.

72. Moore JN, Healy JR, Thoma BN, et al. A population pharmacokinetic model for vancomycin in adult patients receiving extracorporeal membrane oxygenation therapy. CPT Pharmacometrics Syst Pharmacol 2016;5(9):495–502. Available at: http://www.ncbi.nlm.nih.gov/pmc/articles/PMC5036424/.

73. Donadello K, Roberts JA, Cristallini S, et al. Vancomycin population pharmacokinetics during extracorporeal membrane oxygenation therapy: a matched cohort study. Crit Care 2014;18(6):632.

74. Park SJ, Yang JH, Park HJ, et al. Trough concentrations of vancomycin in patients undergoing extracorporeal membrane oxygenation. PLoS One 2015;10(11): e0141016. Available at: http://www.ncbi.nlm.nih.gov/pmc/articles/PMC4636270/.

75. Wu C, Shen L, Hsu L, et al. Pharmacokinetics of vancomycin in adults receiving extracorporeal membrane oxygenation. J Formos Med Assoc 2016;115(7): 560–70.

76. Levison ME, Levison JH. Pharmacokinetics and pharmacodynamics of antibacterial agents. Infect Dis Clin North Am 2009;23(4):791–815, vii.

77. Roberts JA, Lipman J. Pharmacokinetic issues for antibiotics in the critically ill patient. Crit Care Med 2009;37(3):840–51.

78. Welsch C, Augustin P, Allyn J, et al. Alveolar and serum concentrations of imipenem in two lung transplant recipients supported with extracorporeal membrane oxygenation. Transpl Infect Dis 2015;17(1):103–5.

79. Shekar K, Fraser JF, Taccone FS, et al. The combined effects of extracorporeal membrane oxygenation and renal replacement therapy on meropenem pharmacokinetics: a matched cohort study. Crit Care 2014;18(6):565. Available at: http://www.ncbi.nlm.nih.gov/pmc/articles/PMC4302127/.

80. Donadello K, Antonucci E, Cristallini S, et al. β-lactam pharmacokinetics during extracorporeal membrane oxygenation therapy: a case–control study. Int J Antimicrob Agents 2015;45(3):278–82.

81. Gélisse E, Neuville M, de Montmollin E, et al. Extracorporeal membrane oxygenation (ECMO) does not impact on amikacin pharmacokinetics: a case-control study. Intensive Care Med 2016;42(5):946–8.

82. de Montmollin E, Bouadma L, Gault N, et al. Predictors of insufficient amikacin peak concentration in critically ill patients receiving a 25 mg/kg total body weight regimen. Intensive Care Med 2014;40(7):998–1005.
83. Turner RB, Rouse S, Elbarbry F, et al. Azithromycin pharmacokinetics in adults with acute respiratory distress syndrome undergoing treatment with extracorporeal-membrane oxygenation. Ann Pharmacother 2016;50(1):72–3.
84. De Rosa FG, Corcione S, Baietto L, et al. Pharmacokinetics of linezolid during extracorporeal membrane oxygenation. Int J Antimicrob Agents 2013;41(6): 590–1.
85. Veinstein A, Debouverie O, Grégoire N, et al. Lack of effect of extracorporeal membrane oxygenation on tigecycline pharmacokinetics. J Antimicrob Chemother 2012;67(4):1047–8.
86. Pettignano R, Heard MF, Davis RF, et al. Total enteral nutrition versus total parenteral nutrition during pediatric extracorporeal membrane oxygenation. Crit Care Med 1998;26(2):358–63.
87. Flordelis Lasierra JL, Perez-Vela JL, Montejo Gonzalez JC. Enteral nutrition in the hemodynamically unstable critically ill patient. Med Intensiva 2015;39(1):40–8.
88. Mulla H, Peek GJ, Harvey C, et al. Oseltamivir pharmacokinetics in critically ill adults receiving extracorporeal membrane oxygenation support. Anaesth Intensive Care 2013;41(1):66–73.
89. Eyler RF, Heung M, Pleva M, et al. Pharmacokinetics of oseltamivir and oseltamivir carboxylate in critically ill patients receiving continuous venovenous hemodialysis and/or extracorporeal membrane oxygenation. Pharmacotherapy 2012; 32(12):1061–9.
90. Lemaitre F, Luyt CE, Roullet-Renoleau FF, et al. Impact of extracorporeal membrane oxygenation and continuous venovenous hemodiafiltration on the pharmacokinetics of oseltamivir carboxylate in critically ill patients with pandemic (H1N1) influenza. Ther Drug Monit 2012;34(2):171–5.
91. Aebi C, Headrick CL, McCracken GH Jr, et al. Intravenous ribavirin therapy in a neonate with disseminated adenovirus infection undergoing extracorporeal membrane oxygenation: pharmacokinetics and clearance by hemofiltration. J Pediatr 1997;130(4):612–5.
92. Hertzog J, Brackett E, Sale M, et al. Amphotericin B pharmacokinetics during extracorporeal membrane oxygenation: a case report. J Extra Corpor Technol 1996;28(2):94.
93. Ruiz S, Papy E, Da Silva D, et al. Potential voriconazole and caspofungin sequestration during extracorporeal membrane oxygenation. Intensive Care Med 2008; 35(1):183.
94. Spriet I, Annaert P, Meersseman P, et al. Pharmacokinetics of caspofungin and voriconazole in critically ill patients during extracorporeal membrane oxygenation. J Antimicrob Chemother 2009;63(4):767–70.
95. Saini L, Seki JT, Kumar D, et al. Serum voriconazole level variability in patients with hematological malignancies receiving voriconazole therapy. Can J Infect Dis Med Microbiol 2014;25(5):271–6.
96. Strunk A, Ciesek S, Schmidt JJ, et al. Single- and multiple-dose pharmacokinetics of ethambutol and rifampicin in a tuberculosis patient with acute respiratory distress syndrome undergoing extended daily dialysis and ECMO treatment. Int J Infect Dis 2016;42:1–3.

1. Publication Title	2. Publication Number	3. Filing Date
CRITICAL CARE CLINICS	000 – 708	9/18/2017

4. Issue Frequency	5. Number of Issues Published Annually	6. Annual Subscription Price
JAN, APR, JUL, OCT	4	$221.00

7. Complete Mailing Address of Known Office of Publication (Not printer) (Street, city, county, state, and ZIP+4®)

ELSEVIER INC.
230 Park Avenue, Suite 800
New York, NY 10169

Contact Person
STEPHEN R. BUSHING
Telephone (Include area code)
215-239-3688

8. Complete Mailing Address of Headquarters or General Business Office of Publisher (Not printer)

ELSEVIER INC.
230 Park Avenue, Suite 800
New York, NY 10169

9. Full Names and Complete Mailing Addresses of Publisher, Editor, and Managing Editor (Do not leave blank)

Publisher (Name and complete mailing address)

ADRIANNE BRIGIDO, ELSEVIER INC.
1600 JOHN F KENNEDY BLVD. SUITE 1800
PHILADELPHIA, PA 19103-2899

Editor (Name and complete mailing address)

PATRICK MANLEY, ELSEVIER INC.
1600 JOHN F KENNEDY BLVD. SUITE 1800
PHILADELPHIA, PA 19103-2899

Managing Editor (Name and complete mailing address)

PATRICK MANLEY, ELSEVIER INC.
1600 JOHN F KENNEDY BLVD. SUITE 1800
PHILADELPHIA, PA 19103-2899

10. Owner (Do not leave blank. If the publication is owned by a corporation, give the name and address of the corporation immediately followed by the names and addresses of all stockholders owning or holding 1 percent or more of the total amount of stock. If not owned by a corporation, give the names and addresses of the individual owners. If owned by a partnership or other unincorporated firm, give its name and address as well as those of each individual owner. If the publication is published by a nonprofit organization, give its name and address.)

Full Name	Complete Mailing Address
WHOLLY OWNED SUBSIDIARY OF REED/ELSEVIER, US HOLDINGS	1600 JOHN F KENNEDY BLVD. SUITE 1800 PHILADELPHIA, PA 19103-2899

11. Known Bondholders, Mortgagees, and Other Security Holders Owning or Holding 1 Percent or More of Total Amount of Bonds, Mortgages, or Other Securities. If none, check box ▶ ☐ None

Full Name	Complete Mailing Address
N/A	

12. Tax Status (For completion by nonprofit organizations authorized to mail at nonprofit rates) (Check one)
The purpose, function, and nonprofit status of this organization and the exempt status for federal income tax purposes:
☒ Has Not Changed During Preceding 12 Months
☐ Has Changed During Preceding 12 Months (Publisher must submit explanation of change with this statement)

13. Publication Title	14. Issue Date for Circulation Data Below
CRITICAL CARE CLINICS	JULY 2017

15. Extent and Nature of Circulation			Average No. Copies Each Issue During Preceding 12 Months	No. Copies of Single Issue Published Nearest to Filing Date
a. Total Number of Copies (Net press run)			571	415
b. Paid Circulation (By Mail and Outside the Mail)	(1)	Mailed Outside-County Paid Subscriptions Stated on PS Form 3541 (Include paid distribution above nominal rate, advertiser's proof copies, and exchange copies)	277	243
	(2)	Mailed In-County Paid Subscriptions Stated on PS Form 3541 (Include paid distribution above nominal rate, advertiser's proof copies, and exchange copies)	0	0
	(3)	Paid Distribution Outside the Mails Including Sales Through Dealers and Carriers, Street Vendors, Counter Sales, and Other Paid Distribution Outside USPS®	120	103
	(4)	Paid Distribution by Other Classes of Mail Through the USPS (e.g., First-Class Mail®)	0	0
c. Total Paid Distribution (Sum of 15b (1), (2), (3), and (4))			397	346
d. Free or Nominal Rate Distribution (By Mail and Outside the Mail)	(1)	Free or Nominal Rate Outside-County Copies included on PS Form 3541	69	69
	(2)	Free or Nominal Rate In-County Copies included on PS Form 3541	0	0
	(3)	Free or Nominal Rate Copies Mailed at Other Classes Through the USPS (e.g. First-Class Mail)	0	0
	(4)	Free or Nominal Rate Distribution Outside the Mail (Carriers or other means)	0	0
e. Total Free or Nominal Rate Distribution (Sum of 15d (1), (2), (3) and (4))			69	69
f. Total Distribution (Sum of 15c and 15e)			466	415
g. Copies not Distributed (See Instructions to Publishers #4 (page #3))			105	0
h. Total (Sum of 15f and g)			571	415
i. Percent Paid (15c divided by 15f times 100)			85.19%	83.37%

* If you are claiming electronic copies, go to line 16 on page 3. If you are not claiming electronic copies, skip to line 17 on page 3.

16. Electronic Copy Circulation		Average No. Copies Each Issue During Preceding 12 Months	No. Copies of Single Issue Published Nearest to Filing Date
a. Paid Electronic Copies	▶	0	0
b. Total Paid Print Copies (Line 15c) + Paid Electronic Copies (Line 16a)	▶	397	346
c. Total Print Distribution (Line 15f) + Paid Electronic Copies (Line 16a)	▶	466	415
d. Percent Paid (Both Print & Electronic Copies) (16b divided by 16c × 100)	▶	85.19%	83.37%

☒ I certify that 50% of all my distributed copies (electronic and print) are paid above a nominal price.

17. Publication of Statement of Ownership

☒ If the publication is a general publication, publication of this statement is required. Will be printed ☐ Publication not required.
in the OCTOBER 2017 issue of this publication

18. Signature and Title of Editor, Publisher, Business Manager, or Owner

STEPHEN R. BUSHING – INVENTORY DISTRIBUTION CONTROL MANAGER

Date 9/18/2017

I certify that all information furnished on this form is true and complete. I understand that anyone who furnishes false or misleading information on this form or who omits material or information requested on the form may be subject to criminal sanctions (including fines and imprisonment) and/or civil sanctions (including civil penalties).

Moving?

Make sure your subscription moves with you!

To notify us of your new address, find your **Clinics Account Number** (located on your mailing label above your name), and contact customer service at:

Email: journalscustomerservice-usa@elsevier.com

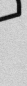

800-654-2452 (subscribers in the U.S. & Canada)
314-447-8871 (subscribers outside of the U.S. & Canada)

Fax number: 314-447-8029

Elsevier Health Sciences Division
Subscription Customer Service
3251 Riverport Lane
Maryland Heights, MO 63043

*To ensure uninterrupted delivery of your subscription, please notify us at least 4 weeks in advance of move.

ELSEVIER

Printed and bound by CPI Group (UK) Ltd, Croydon, CR0 4YY

03/10/2024

01040390-0014